ASIAN COOKBOOK 2022

QUICK AND EASY AUTHENTIC RECIPES
FOR ABSOLUTE BEGINNERS

CHEN ZENFREN

Table of Contents

Introduction *10*
   Asparagus with Mushrooms and Spring Onions *11*
   Asparagus Stir-Fry *12*
   Sweet and Sour Asparagus *12*
   Aubergine with Basil *13*
   Braised Aubergine *14*
   Braised Aubergine with Tomatoes *15*
   Steamed Aubergine *16*
   Stuffed Aubergine *17*
   Stir-Fried Aubergine *18*
   Bamboo Shoots with Chicken *19*
   Deep-Fried Bamboo Shoots *20*
   Fried Bamboo Shoots *21*
   Bamboo Shoots with Mushrooms *22*
   Bamboo Shoots with Dried Mushrooms *23*
   Bamboo Shoots in Oyster Sauce *24*
   Bamboo Shoots with Sesame Oil *25*
   Bamboo Shoots with Spinach *26*
   Broad Bean Sauté *27*
   Green Beans with Chilli *28*
   Spiced Green Beans *29*
   Stir-Fried Green Beans *29*
   Sautéed Bean Sprouts *30*
   Bean Sprout Stir-Fry *31*
   Bean Sprouts and Celery *32*
   Bean Sprouts and Peppers *33*
   Bean Sprouts with Pork *34*
   Broccoli Stir-Fry *35*
   Broccoli in Brown Sauce *36*
   Cabbage with Bacon Shreds *37*
   Creamed Cabbage *38*
   Chinese Cabbage with Mushrooms *39*

Spicy Cabbage Stir-Fry	40
Sweet and Sour Cabbage	41
Sweet and Sour Red Cabbage	42
Crispy Seaweed	43
Carrots with Honey	44
Carrot and Pepper Stir-Fry	45
Stir-Fried Cauliflower	46
Cauliflower with Mushrooms	47
Celery Stir-Fry	48
Celery and Mushrooms	49
Stir-Fried Chinese Leaves	50
Chinese Leaves in Milk	51
Chinese Leaves with Mushrooms	52
Chinese Leaves with Scallops	53
Steamed Chinese Leaves	54
Chinese Leaves with Water Chestnuts	55
Courgette Stir-Fry	56
Courgettes in Black Bean Sauce	57
Stuffed Courgette Bites	58
Cucumber with Prawns	59
Cucumbers with Sesame Oil	60
Stuffed Cucumbers	61
Stir-Fried Dandelion Leaves	62
Braised Lettuce	63
Stir-Fried Lettuce with Ginger	64
Mangetout with Bamboo Shoots	65
Mangetout with Mushrooms and Ginger	66
Chinese Marrow	67
Stuffed Marrow	68
Mushrooms with Anchovy Sauce	69
Mushrooms and Bamboo Shoots	70
Mushrooms with Bamboo Shoots and Mangetout	71
Mushrooms with Mangetout	72
Spicy Mushrooms	73
Steamed Mushrooms	74
Steamed Stuffed Mushrooms	75

Straw Mushrooms in Oyster Sauce 76
Baked Onions 77
Curried Onions with Peas 78
Pearl Onions in Orange-Ginger Sauce 79
Onion Custard 80
Pak Choi 81
Peas with Mushrooms 82
Stir-Fried Peppers 83
Pepper and Bean Stir-Fry 84
Fish-Stuffed Peppers 85
Pork-Stuffed Peppers 86
Vegetable-Stuffed Peppers 88
Deep-Fried Potatoes and Carrots 89
Potato Sauté 90
Spiced Potatoes 91
Pumpkin with Rice Noodles 92
Shallots in Malt Beer 93
Spinach with Garlic 94
Spinach with Mushrooms 95
Spinach with Ginger 96
Spinach with Peanuts 97
Vegetable Chow Mein 98
Mixed Vegetables 99
Mixed Vegetables with Ginger 100
Vegetable Spring Rolls 101
Simple Stir-Fried Vegetables 103
Vegetables with Honey 104
Fried Spring Vegetables 105
Marinated Steamed Vegetables 107
Vegetable Surprises 108
Sweet and Sour Mixed Vegetables 110
Vegetables in Tomato Sauce 111
Water Chestnut Cakes 113
Simple Chicken Stir-Fry 115
Chicken in Tomato Sauce 116
Chicken with Tomatoes 117

Poached Chicken with Tomatoes	117
Chicken and Tomatoes with Black Bean Sauce	119
Quick-Cooked Chicken with Vegetables	120
Walnut Chicken	121
Chicken with Walnuts	122
Chicken with Water Chestnuts	123
Savoury Chicken with Water Chestnuts	124
Chicken Wontons	125
Crispy Chicken Wings	126
Five-Spice Chicken Wings	127
Marinated Chicken Wings	128
Royal Chicken Wings	130
Spiced Chicken Wings	131
Barbecued Chicken Drumsticks	132
Hoisin Chicken Drumsticks	133
Braised Chicken	134
Crispy-Fried Chicken	135
Deep-Fried Whole Chicken	136
Five-Spice Chicken	137
Ginger and Spring Onion Chicken	139
Poached Chicken	140
Red-Cooked Chicken	141
Red-Cooked Spiced Chicken	142
Sesame Roast Chicken	143
Chicken in Soy Sauce	144
Steamed Chicken	145
Steamed Chicken with Anise	146
Strange-Flavoured Chicken	147
Crispy Chicken Chunks	148
Chicken with Green Beans	149
Cooked Chicken with Pineapple	150
Chicken with Peppers and Tomatoes	151
Sesame Chicken	152
Fried Poussins	153
Turkey with Mangetout	154
Turkey with Peppers	156

Chinese Roast Turkey...158
Turkey with Walnuts and Mushrooms..159
Duck with Bamboo Shoots..160
Duck with Bean Sprouts 161
Braised Duck 162
Steamed Duck with Celery 163
Duck with Ginger...164
Duck with Green Beans..165
Deep-Fried Steamed Duck 166
Duck with Exotic Fruits..167
Braised Duck with Chinese Leaves...169
Drunken Duck...170
Five-Spice Duck...171
Stir-Fried Duck with Ginger 172
Duck with Ham and Leeks 173
Honey-Roast Duck 174
Moist Roast Duck...175
Stir-Fried Duck with Mushrooms 176
Duck with Two Mushrooms 178
Braised Duck with Onions..179
Duck with Orange 181
Orange-Roast Duck..182
Duck with Pears and Chestnuts 183
Peking Duck...184
Braised Duck with Pineapple 186
Stir-Fried Duck with Pineapple 187
Pineapple and Ginger Duck 188
Duck with Pineapple and Lychees 189
Duck with Pork and Chestnuts 190
Duck with Potatoes 191
Red-Cooked Duck 193
Rice Wine Roast Duck..194
Steamed Duck with Rice Wine 195
Savoury Duck..196
Savoury Duck with Green Beans 197
Slow-Cooked Duck..198

Stir-Fried Duck 200
Duck with Sweet Potatoes 201
Sweet and Sour Duck 203
Tangerine Duck 204
Duck with Vegetables 205
Stir-Fried Duck with Vegetables 207
White-Cooked Duck 208
Duck with Wine 209
Wine-Vapour Duck 210
Fried Pheasant 211
Pheasant with Almonds 212
Venison with Dried Mushrooms 213
Salted Eggs 214
Soy Eggs 215
Tea Eggs 216
Egg Custard 217
Steamed Eggs 218

Introduction

Everyone who loves to cook, loves to experiment with new dishes and new taste sensations. Chinese cuisine has become immensely popular in recent years because it offers a different range of flavours to enjoy. Most dishes are cooked on top of the stove, and many are quickly prepared and cooked so are ideal for the busy cook who wants to create an appetising and attractive dish when there is little time to spare. If you really enjoy Chinese cooking, you will probably already have a wok, and this is the perfect utensil for cooking most of the dishes in the book. If you have yet to be convinced that this style of cooking is for you, use a good frying pan or saucepan to try out the recipes. When you find how easy they are to prepare and how tasty to eat, you will almost certainly want to invest in a wok for your kitchen.

Asparagus with Mushrooms and Spring Onions

Serves 4

10 dried Chinese mushrooms
225 g/8 oz asparagus
1 bunch spring onions (scallions), trimmed
600 ml/1 pt/2½ cups chicken stock
5 ml/1 tsp cornflour (cornstarch)
15 ml/1 tbsp water
5 ml/1 tsp salt

Soak the mushrooms in warm water for 30 minutes then drain. Discard the stalks. Arrange the mushrooms in the centre of a strainer then arrange the spring onions and asparagus in a circle radiating out from the centre. Bring the stock to the boil then lower the strainer into the stock, cover and simmer gently for about 10 minutes until the vegetables are just tender. Remove the vegetables and invert them on to a warmed serving plate to maintain the pattern. Bring the stock to the boil. Blend the water, cornflour and salt to a paste, stir it into the stock and simmer, stirring, until the sauce thickens slightly. Spoon over the vegetables and serve at once.

Asparagus Stir-Fry

Serves 4

45 ml/3 tbsp groundnut (peanut) oil
1 spring onion (scallion), chopped
450 g/1 lb asparagus
30 ml/2 tbsp soy sauce
5 ml/1 tsp sugar
120 ml/4 fl oz/½ cup chicken stock
5 ml/1 tsp cornflour (cornstarch)

Heat the oil and fry the spring onion until lightly browned. Add the asparagus and stir-fry for 3 minutes. Add the remaining ingredients and stir-fry for 4 minutes.

Sweet and Sour Asparagus

Serves 4

30 ml/2 tbsp groundnut (peanut) oil
450 g/1 lb asparagus, cut in diagonal pieces
60 ml/4 tbsp wine vinegar
50 g/2 oz/¼ cup brown sugar
15 ml/1 tbsp soy sauce
15 ml/1 tbsp rice wine or dry sherry
5 ml/1 tsp salt

15 ml/1 tbsp cornflour (cornstarch)

Heat the oil and stir-fry the asparagus for 4 minutes. Add the wine vinegar, sugar, soy sauce, wine or sherry and salt and stir-fry for 2 minutes. Mix the cornflour with a little water, stir it into the pan and stir-fry for 1 minute.

Aubergine with Basil

Serves 4

60 ml/4 tbsp groundnut (peanut) oil
2 aubergines (eggplants)
60 ml/4 tbsp water
2 cloves garlic, crushed
1 red chilli pepper, diagonally sliced
45 ml/3 tbsp soy sauce
1 large bunch basil

Heat the oil and fry the aubergine until lightly browned. Add the water, garlic, chilli pepper and soy sauce and stir-fry until the aubergine changes colour. Add the basil and stir-fry until the leaves are wilted. Serve at once.

Braised Aubergine

Serves 4

1 aubergine (eggplant)
oil for deep-frying
15 ml/1 tbsp groundnut (peanut) oil
3 spring onions (scallions), chopped
1 slice ginger root, chopped
90 ml/6 tbsp chicken stock
15 ml/1 tbsp rice wine or dry sherry
15 ml/1 tbsp soy sauce
15 ml/1 tbsp black bean sauce
15 ml/1 tbsp brown sugar

Peel the aubergine and cut it into large cubes. Heat the oil and deep-fry the aubergine until soft and lightly browned. Remove and drain well.

Heat the oil and fry the spring onions and ginger until lightly browned. Add the aubergine and stir well. Add the stock, wine or sherry, soy sauce, black bean sauce and sugar. Stir-fry for 2 minutes.

Braised Aubergine with Tomatoes

Serves 4

6 slices bacon

2 cloves garlic, crushed

2 spring onions (scallions), chopped

1 aubergine (eggplant), peeled and diced

4 tomatoes, skinned and quartered

salt and freshly ground pepper

Cut the rind off the bacon and cut into chunks. Fry until lightly browned. Add the garlic and spring onions and stir-fry for 2 minutes. Add the aubergine and stir-fry for about 5 minutes until slightly soft. Carefully mix in the tomatoes and season with salt and pepper. Stir gently over a low heat until heated through.

Steamed Aubergine

Serves 4

1 aubergine (eggplant)
30 ml/2 tbsp soy sauce
5 ml/1 tsp groundnut (peanut) oil

Score the aubergine skin a few times and place it in an ovenproof dish. Place on a rack in a steamer and steam over gently simmering water for about 25 minutes until soft. Leave to cool slightly then peel off the skin and tear the flesh into shreds. Sprinkle with soy sauce and oil and stir well. Serve hot or cold.

Stuffed Aubergine

Serves 4

4 dried Chinese mushrooms
225 g/8 oz minced (ground) pork
2 spring onions (scallions), minced
1 slice ginger root, minced
30 ml/2 tbsp soy sauce
15 ml/1 tbsp rice wine or dry sherry
5 ml/1 tsp sugar
1 aubergine (eggplant), halved lengthways

Soak the mushrooms in warm water for 30 minutes then drain. Discard the stalks and chop the caps. Mix with the pork, spring onions, ginger, soy sauce, wine or sherry and sugar. Scoop out the seeds of the aubergine to make a hollow shape. Stuff with the pork mixture and arrange in an ovenproof dish. Place on a rack in a steamer and steam over gently simmering water for 30 minutes until tender.

Stir-Fried Aubergine

Serves 4–6

4 dried Chinese mushrooms
1 aubergine (eggplant), peeled and diced
30 ml/2 tbsp cornflour (cornstarch)
oil for deep-frying
45 ml/3 tbsp groundnut (peanut) oil
50 g/2 oz cooked chicken, diced
50 g/2 oz smoked ham, diced
50 g/2 oz bamboo shoots, chopped
50 g/2 oz/½ cup chopped mixed nuts
5 ml/1 tsp salt
5 ml/1 tsp sugar
30 ml/2 tbsp soy sauce
30 ml/2 tbsp rice wine or dry sherry

Soak the mushrooms in warm water for 30 minutes then drain. Discard the stalks and slice the caps. Toss the aubergine lightly in cornflour. Heat the oil and deep-fry the aubergine until golden. Remove from the pan and drain well. Heat the oil and stir-fry the chicken, ham, bamboo shoots and nuts. Add the remaining ingredients and stir-fry for 3 minutes. Return the aubergine to the pan and stir-fry until heated through.

Bamboo Shoots with Chicken

Serves 4

50 g/2 oz chicken meat, minced (ground)
50 g/2 oz smoked ham, minced (ground)
50 g/2 oz water chestnuts, minced (ground)
2 egg whites
15 ml/1 tbsp cornflour (cornstarch)
225 g/8 oz bamboo shoots, cut into thick strips
15 ml/1 tbsp chopped flat-leaved parsley

Mix together the chicken, ham and water chestnuts. Mix together the egg whites and cornflour then stir them into the minced ingredients. Stir the bamboo shoots into the mixture until well coated then arrange in an ovenproof dish. Place on a rack in a steamer, cover and steam over gently simmering water for 15 minutes. Serve garnished with parsley.

Deep-Fried Bamboo Shoots

Serves 4

oil for deep-frying
225 g/8 oz bamboo shoots, cut into strips
15 ml/1 tbsp groundnut (peanut) oil
15 ml/1 tbsp brown sugar
15 ml/1 tbsp soy sauce
10 ml/2 tsp cornflour (cornstarch)
90 ml/6 tbsp water

Heat the oil and deep-fry the bamboo shoots until golden. Drain well. Heat the groundnut (peanut) oil and stir-fry the bamboo shoots until coated with oil. Mix together the sugar, soy sauce, cornflour and water, stir into the pan and stir-fry until heated through.

Fried Bamboo Shoots

Serves 4

90 ml/6 tbsp groundnut (peanut) oil

1 spring onion, cut into strips

1 clove garlic, crushed

1 red chilli pepper, cut into strips

225 g/8 oz bamboo shoots

15 ml/1 tbsp thick soy sauce

2.5 ml/½ tsp sesame oil

Heat the oil and stir-fry the spring onion, garlic and chilli pepper for 30 seconds. Add the bamboo shoots and stir-fry until just tender and well coated in the spices. Add the soy sauce and sesame oil and stir-fry for a further 3 minutes. Serve at once.

Bamboo Shoots with Mushrooms

Serves 4

8 dried Chinese mushrooms

45 ml/3 tbsp groundnut (peanut) oil

350 g/12 oz bamboo shoots, cut into strips

30 ml/2 tbsp soy sauce

5 ml/1 tsp brown sugar

15 ml/1 tbsp cornflour (cornstarch)

45 ml/3 tbsp water

Soak the mushrooms in warm water for 30 minutes then drain. Discard the stalks and slice the caps. Heat the oil and stir-fry the mushrooms for 2 minutes. Add the bamboo shoots and stir-fry for 3 minutes. Add the soy sauce and sugar and stir well until heated through. Transfer the vegetables to a warmed serving plate using a slotted spoon. Mix the cornflour and water to a paste and stir it into the pan. Simmer, stirring, until the sauce clears and thickens then pour it over the vegetables and serve at once.

Bamboo Shoots with Dried Mushrooms

Serves 4

6 dried Chinese mushrooms
250 ml/8 fl oz/1 cup chicken stock
15 ml/1 tbsp rice wine or dry sherry
15 ml/1 tbsp soy sauce
15 ml/1 tbsp groundnut (peanut) oil
225 g/8 oz bamboo shoots, sliced
15 ml/1 tbsp cornflour (cornstarch)

Soak the mushrooms in warm water for 30 minutes then drain. Discard the stems and slice the caps. Place the mushroom caps in a pan with half the stock, the wine or sherry and soy sauce. Bring to the boil, cover and simmer for about 10 minutes until thick. Add the oil and stir over a medium heat for 2 minutes. Add the bamboo shoots and stir-fry for 3 minutes. Mix the cornflour into the remaining stock and stir it into the pan. Bring to the boil, stirring, then simmer for about 4 minutes until the sauce thickens and clears.

Bamboo Shoots in Oyster Sauce

Serves 4

15 ml/1 tbsp groundnut (peanut) oil
350 g/12 oz bamboo shoots, cut into strips
250 ml/8 fl oz/1 cup chicken stock
15 ml/1 tbsp oyster sauce
5 ml/1 tsp soy sauce
2.5 ml/½ tsp brown sugar
2.5 ml/½ tsp sesame oil

Heat the oil and stir-fry the bamboo shoots for 1 minute. Add the stock, oyster sauce, soy sauce and sugar and bring to the boil. Simmer for about 10 minutes until the bamboo shoots are tender and the liquid has reduced. Serve sprinkled with sesame oil.

Bamboo Shoots with Sesame Oil

Serves 4

100 g/4 oz bean sprouts

45 ml/3 tbsp groundnut (peanut) oil

225 g/8 oz bamboo shoots

5 ml/1 tsp salt

5 ml/1 tsp sesame oil

Cook the bean sprouts in boiling water for about 10 minutes until tender but still crisp. Drain well. Meanwhile, heat the oil and stir-fry the bamboo shoots for about 5 minutes until tender but still crisp. Sprinkle with salt, mix well then arrange with the bean sprouts on a warmed serving plate. Sprinkle with sesame oil and serve.

Bamboo Shoots with Spinach

Serves 4

45 ml/3 tbsp groundnut (peanut) oil
450 g/1 lb bamboo shoots
5 ml/1 tsp rice wine or dry sherry
pinch of salt
120 ml/4 fl oz/½ cup chicken stock
100 g/4 oz spinach
2.5 ml/½ tsp sesame oil

Heat the oil and fry the bamboo shoots for about 1 minute. Add the wine or sherry, salt and stock, bring to the boil and simmer for 3 minutes. Add the spinach and simmer until the spinach has wilted and the liquid reduced slightly. Transfer to a warmed serving bowl and serve sprinkled with sesame oil.

Broad Bean Sauté

Serves 4

450 g/1 lb shelled broad beans
60 ml/4 tbsp groundnut (peanut) oil
5 ml/1 tsp salt
10 ml/2 tsp brown sugar
75 ml/5 tbsp chicken stock
salt
2 spring onions (scallions), chopped

Place the beans in a pan, just cover with water, bring to the boil and simmer until tender. Drain well.

Heat the oil then add the beans and stir until well coated with oil. Add the sugar and stock and season to taste with salt. Stir-fry for 3 minutes. Stir in the spring onions and serve.

Green Beans with Chilli

Serves 4

45 ml/3 tbsp groundnut (peanut) oil
2 dried red chilli peppers
2 onions, chopped
450 g/1 lb green beans

Heat the oil with the chilli peppers and fry until they change colour then remove them from the pan. Add the onions and stir-fry until lightly browned. Meanwhile, blanch the beans in boiling water for 2 minutes then drain well. Add to the onions and stir-fry for 10 minutes until tender but still crisp and well coated in the spiced oil.

Spiced Green Beans

Serves 4

450 g/1 lb green beans
15 ml/1 tbsp salt
5 ml/1 tsp ground anise
5 ml/1 tsp freshly ground red pepper

Place all the ingredients in a large pan and just cover with water. Bring to the boil and simmer for about 8 minutes until the beans are just tender. Drain well before serving.

Stir-Fried Green Beans

Serves 4

45 ml/3 tbsp groundnut (peanut) oil
5 ml/1 tsp salt
450 g/1 lb string beans, cut into pieces
120 ml/4 fl oz/½ cup chicken stock
15 ml/1 tbsp soy sauce

Heat the oil and salt then add the beans and stir-fry for 2 minutes. Add the stock and soy sauce, bring to the boil, cover and simmer for about 5 minutes until the beans are tender but still slightly crisp.

Sautéed Bean Sprouts

Serves 4

15 ml/1 tbsp groundnut (peanut) oil
450 g/1 lb bean sprouts
15 ml/1 tbsp soy sauce
salt and freshly ground pepper

Heat the oil and stir-fry the bean sprouts for about 3 minutes. Add the soy sauce, salt and pepper and stir together well. Cover and simmer for 5 minutes then remove the lid and simmer for a further 1 minute.

Bean Sprout Stir-Fry

Serves 4

15 ml/1 tbsp groundnut (peanut) oil

2.5 ml/½ tsp salt

1 clove garlic, crushed

450 g/1 lb bean sprouts

3 spring onions (scallions), chopped

60 ml/4 tbsp chicken stock

5 ml/1 tsp sugar

5 ml/1 tsp soy sauce

Heat the oil, salt and garlic until the garlic turns light golden. Add the bean sprouts and spring onions and stir-fry for 2 minutes. Add the remaining ingredients and stir-fry for a few minutes until all the liquid has evaporated.

Bean Sprouts and Celery

Serves 4

450 g/1 lb bean sprouts

45 ml/3 tbsp groundnut (peanut) oil

4 stalks celery, cut into strips

5 ml/1 tsp salt

15 ml/1 tbsp soy sauce

90 ml/6 tbsp chicken stock

Blanch the bean sprouts in boiling water for 3 minutes then drain. Heat the oil and stir-fry the celery for 1 minute. Add the bean sprouts and stir-fry for 1 minute. Add the remaining ingredients, bring to the boil, cover and simmer for 3 minutes before serving.

Bean Sprouts and Peppers

Serves 4

225 g/8 oz bean sprouts

45 ml/3 tbsp groundnut (peanut) oil

2 dried chilli peppers

1 slice ginger root, minced

1 red pepper, cut into strips

1 green pepper, cut into strips

90 ml/6 tbsp chicken stock

Blanch the bean sprouts in boiling water for 3 minutes then drain. Heat the oil and fry the whole chilli peppers for about 3 minutes then discard the peppers. Add the ginger and peppers to the pan and stir-fry for 3 minutes. Add the bean sprouts and stir-fry for 2 minutes. Add the stock, bring to the boil, cover and simmer for 3 minutes before serving.

Bean Sprouts with Pork

Serves 4

450 g/1 lb bean sprouts

100 g/4 oz lean pork, cut into strips

15 ml/1 tbsp cornflour (cornstarch)

15 ml/1 tbsp rice wine

15 ml/1 tbsp soy sauce

5 ml/1 tsp sugar

2.5 ml/½ tsp salt

30 ml/2 tbsp groundnut (peanut) oil

75 ml/5 tbsp chicken stock

Blanch the bean sprouts in boiling water for 3 minutes then drain. Toss the pork with the cornflour, wine or sherry, soy sauce, sugar and salt then leave to stand for 30 minutes. Heat half the oil and stir-fry the bean sprouts for 1 minute. Remove from the pan. Heat the remaining oil and stir-fry the pork until lightly browned. Add the stock, cover and simmer for 3 minutes. Return the bean sprouts to the pan and stir until heated through. Serve at once.

Broccoli Stir-Fry

Serves 4

45 ml/3 tbsp groundnut (peanut) oil

1 spring onion (scallion), chopped

450 g/1 lb broccoli florets

30 ml/2 tbsp soy sauce

5 ml/1 tsp sugar

120 ml/4 fl oz/½ cup chicken stock

5 ml/1 tsp cornflour (cornstarch)

Heat the oil and fry the spring onion until lightly browned. Add the broccoli and stir-fry for 3 minutes. Add the remaining ingredients and stir-fry for 2 minutes.

Broccoli in Brown Sauce

Serves 4

225 g/8 oz broccoli florets
30 ml/2 tbsp groundnut (peanut) oil
1 clove garlic, crushed
100 g/4 oz bamboo shoots, sliced
250 ml/8 fl oz/1 cup chicken stock
15 ml/1 tbsp soy sauce
15 ml/1 tbsp oyster sauce
15 ml/1 tbsp cornflour (cornstarch)
30 ml/2 tbsp rice wine or dry sherry

Parboil the broccoli in boiling water for 4 minutes then drain well. Heat the oil and fry the garlic until golden brown. Add the broccoli and bamboo shoots and stir-fry for 1 minute. Add the stock, soy sauce and oyster sauce, bring to the boil, cover and simmer for 4 minutes. Mix the cornflour and wine or sherry, stir it into the pan and simmer, stirring, until the sauce has thickened.

Cabbage with Bacon Shreds

Serves 4

350 g/12 oz cabbage, finely shredded
salt
3 slices streaky bacon, rinded and cut into strips
30 ml/2 tbsp groundnut (peanut) oil
2 cloves garlic
5 ml/1 tsp grated ginger root
5 ml/1 tsp sugar
120 ml/4 fl oz/½ cup chicken or vegetable stock

Sprinkle the cabbage with salt and leave to stand for 15 minutes. Fry the bacon until crisp. Heat the oil and fry the garlic until lightly browned then discard. Add the cabbage to the pan with the ginger and sugar and stir-fry for 2 minutes. Add the stock and bacon and stir-fry for a further 2 minutes. Serve with fried rice.

Creamed Cabbage

Serves 4

450 g/1 lb Chinese cabbage

45 ml/3 tbsp groundnut (peanut) oil

250 ml/8 fl oz/1 cup chicken stock

salt

15 ml/1 tbsp cornflour (cornstarch)

50 g/2 oz smoked ham, diced

Cut the cabbage into 5 cm/2 in strips. Heat the oil and stir-fry the cabbage for 3 minutes. Add the stock and season with salt. Bring to the boil, cover and simmer for 4 minutes. Mix the cornflour with a little water, stir it into the pan and simmer, stirring, until the sauce thickens. Transfer to a warmed serving plate and serve sprinkled with ham.

Chinese Cabbage with Mushrooms

Serves 4

6 dried Chinese mushrooms
45 ml/3 tbsp groundnut (peanut) oil
1 Chinese cabbage, diced
1 red pepper, diced
1 green pepper, diced
225 g/8 oz garlic sausage, diced
120 ml/4 fl oz/½ cup chicken stock
45 ml/3 tbsp wine vinegar
20 ml/4 tsp soy sauce
20 ml/4 tsp honey
5 ml/1 tsp cornflour (cornstarch)
salt and freshly ground pepper
20 ml/2 tbsp chopped chives

Soak the mushrooms in warm water for 30 minutes then drain. Discard the stalks and chop the caps. Heat the oil and stir-fry the mushrooms, cabbage and peppers for 5 minutes. Add the garlic sausage and fry briefly. Mix the stock with the wine vinegar, soy sauce, honey and cornflour. Stir into the pan and bring to the boil. Season with salt and pepper and simmer, stirring, until the sauce thickens. Serve sprinkled with chives.

Spicy Cabbage Stir-Fry

Serves 4

450 g/1 lb cabbage, shredded

30 ml/2 tbsp groundnut (peanut) oil

2 cloves garlic, crushed

1 slice ginger root, minced

15 ml/1 tbsp oyster sauce

15 ml/1 tbsp soy sauce

15 ml/1 tbsp chilli bean sauce

5 ml/1 tsp sesame oil

Blanch the cabbage in boiling salted water for 2 minutes. Drain well. Heat the oil and stir-fry the garlic and ginger for a few seconds until lightly browned. Add the cabbage and stir-fry for 2 minutes. Add the remaining ingredients and stir-fry for a further 2 minutes.

Sweet and Sour Cabbage

Serves 4

15 ml/1 tbsp groundnut (peanut) oil

1 head cabbage, shredded

5 ml/1 tsp salt

30 ml/2 tbsp wine vinegar

30 ml/2 tbsp sugar

15 ml/1 tbsp soy sauce

15 ml/1 tbsp cornflour (cornstarch)

45 ml/3 tbsp water

Heat the oil and stir-fry the cabbage for 3 minutes. Add the salt and continue to stir-fry until the cabbage is just tender. Blend the wine vinegar, sugar, soy sauce, cornflour and water to a paste, add it to the pan and simmer, stirring, until the sauce coats the cabbage.

Sweet and Sour Red Cabbage

Serves 4

30 ml/2 tbsp groundnut (peanut) oil

450 g/1 lb red cabbage, shredded

50 g/2 oz/¼ cup brown sugar

45 ml/ 3 tbsp wine vinegar

15 ml/1 tbsp soy sauce

5 ml/ 1 tsp salt

15 ml/1 tbsp cornflour (cornstarch)

Heat the oil and stir-fry the cabbage for 4 minutes. Add the sugar, wine vinegar, soy sauce and salt and stir-fry for 2 minutes. Mix the cornflour with a little water and stir-fry for 1 minute.

Crispy Seaweed

Serves 4

750 g/1½ lb spring greens, very finely shredded
oil for deep-frying
5 ml/1 tsp salt
10 ml/2 tsp caster sugar

Rinse the greens then dry thoroughly. Heat the oil and deep-fry the greens in batches over a medium heat until they float to the surface. Remove from the oil and drain well on kitchen paper. Sprinkle with salt and sugar and toss together gently. Serve cold.

Carrots with Honey

Serves 4

1 kg/2 lb small spring carrots

20 ml/4 tsp groundnut (peanut) oil

20 ml/4 tsp unsalted butter

15 ml/1 tbsp water

10 ml/2 tsp honey

15 ml/1 tbsp chopped fresh coriander

100 g/4 oz pine kernels

salt and freshly ground pepper

Wash the carrots and cut the green down to 5 mm/¼ in. Heat the oil and butter, add the water and honey and bring to the boil. Add the carrots and cook for about 4 minutes. Add the coriander and pine kernels and season with salt and pepper.

Carrot and Pepper Stir-Fry

Serves 4

30 ml/2 tbsp groundnut (peanut) oil

2.5 ml/½ tsp salt

4 carrots, sliced

1 green pepper, cut into strips

30 ml/2 tbsp sugar

15 ml/1 tbsp wine vinegar

250 ml/8 fl oz/1 cup chicken tock

15 ml/1 tbsp cornflour (cornstarch)

Heat the oil and salt then add the carrots and pepper and stir-fry for 3 minutes. Add the sugar, wine vinegar and half the stock, bring to the boil, cover and simmer for 5 minutes. Stir the cornflour into the remaining stock, add to the pan and simmer, stirring, until the sauce thickens and clears.

Stir-Fried Cauliflower

Serves 4

450 g/1 lb cauliflower florets
45 ml/3 tbsp groundnut (peanut) oil
1 spring onion (scallion), chopped
120 ml/4 fl oz/½ cup chicken stock
5 ml/1 tsp cornflour (cornstarch)

Blanch the cauliflower in boiling water for 2 minutes then drain well. Heat the oil and fry the spring onion until lightly browned. Add the cauliflower and stir-fry for 4 minutes. Add the remaining ingredients and stir-fry for 2 minutes.

Cauliflower with Mushrooms

Serves 4

6 dried Chinese mushrooms
1 small cauliflower
45 ml/3 tbsp groundnut (peanut) oil
100 g/4 oz water chestnuts, sliced
45 ml/3 tbsp soy sauce
15 ml/1 tbsp rice wine or dry sherry
5 ml/1 tsp cornflour (cornstarch)
30 ml/2 tbsp water

Soak the mushrooms in warm water for 30 minutes then drain, reserving 120 ml/4 fl oz/½ cup of liquid. Discard the stalks and slice the caps. Cut the cauliflower into small florets. Heat the oil and stir-fry the mushrooms until coated with oil. Add the water chestnuts and stir-fry for 1 minute. Mix the soy sauce and wine or sherry with the mushroom liquid and add it to the pan with the cauliflower. Bring to the boil, cover and simmer for 5 minutes. Blend the cornflour and water to a paste, stir into the sauce and simmer, stirring, until the sauce thickens.

Celery Stir-Fry

Serves 4

30 ml/2 tbsp groundnut (peanut) oil
6 spring onions (scallions), chopped
½ head celery, cut into chunks
15 ml/1 tbsp soy sauce
5 ml/1 tsp salt

Heat the oil and fry the spring onions until lightly browned. Add the celery and stir until well coated with oil. Add the soy sauce and salt, stir well, cover and simmer for 3 minutes.

Celery and Mushrooms

Serves 4

45 ml/3 tbsp groundnut (peanut) oil
6 stalks celery, diagonally sliced
225 g/8 oz mushrooms, sliced
30 ml/2 tbsp rice wine or dry sherry
salt and freshly ground pepper

Heat the oil and stir-fry the celery for 3 minutes. Add the mushrooms and stir-fry for 2 minutes. Add the wine or sherry and season with salt and pepper. Stir-fry for a few minutes until heated through.

Stir-Fried Chinese Leaves

Serves 4

15 ml/1 tbsp groundnut (peanut) oil
1 clove garlic, chopped
3 spring onions (scallions), chopped
350 g/12 oz Chinese leaves, shredded
2.5 ml/½ tsp salt
450 ml/¾ pt boiling water

Heat the oil and fry the garlic and onion until lightly browned. Add the Chinese leaves and salt and stir well. Add the boiling water, return to the boil, cover arid simmer for about 5 minutes until the Chinese leaves are tender but still crisp. Drain well.

Chinese Leaves in Milk

Serves 4

350 g/12 oz Chinese leaves, shredded

45 ml/3 tbsp groundnut (peanut) oil

3 spring onions (scallions), chopped

15 ml/1 tbsp rice wine or dry sherry

90 ml/6 tbsp chicken stock

salt

90 ml/6 tbsp milk

15 ml/1 tbsp cornflour (cornstarch)

5 ml/1 tsp sesame oil

Steam the Chinese leaves for about 5 minutes until just tender. Heat the oil and fry the spring onions until lightly browned. Add the wine or sherry and chicken stock and season with salt. Stir in the cabbage, cover and simmer gently for 5 minutes. Mix the milk and cornflour, stir into pan and simmer, stirring, for 2 minutes. Serve sprinkled with sesame oil.

Chinese Leaves with Mushrooms

Serves 4

50 g/2 oz dried Chinese mushrooms
450 g/1 lb Chinese leaves
45 ml/3 tbsp groundnut (peanut) oil
120 ml/4 fl oz/½ cup chicken stock
15 ml/1 tbsp soy sauce
5 ml/1 tsp salt
5 ml/1 tsp sugar
15 ml/1 tbsp cornflour (cornstarch)
10 ml/2 tsp sesame oil

Soak the mushrooms in warm water for 30 minutes then drain. Discard the stems and slice the caps. Cut the head of Chinese leaves into thick slices. Heat half the oil, add the Chinese leaves and stir-fry for 2 minutes. Add the chicken stock, soy sauce, salt and sugar and stir-fry for about 4 minutes. Add the mushrooms and stir-fry until the vegetables are tender. Mix the cornflour with a little water, stir it into the sauce and simmer, stirring until the sauce clears and thickens. Serve sprinkled with sesame oil.

Chinese Leaves with Scallops

Serves 4

4 hearts Chinese leaves
600 ml/1 pt/2½ cups chicken stock
100 g/4 oz shelled scallops, sliced
5 ml/1 tsp cornflour (cornstarch)

Place the Chinese leaves and stock in a pan, bring to the boil and simmer for about 10 minutes until just tender. Transfer the Chinese leaves to a warmed serving plate and keep them warm. Pour out all but 250 ml/8 fl oz/1 cup of the stock. Add the scallops and simmer for a few minutes until the scallops are tender. Blend the cornflour with a little water, stir it into the pan and simmer, stirring, until the sauce thickens slightly. Pour over the Chinese leaves and serve.

Steamed Chinese Leaves

Serves 4

450 g/1 lb Chinese leaves, separated
15 ml/1 tbsp cornflour (cornstarch)
5 ml/1 tsp salt
300 ml/½ pt/1¼ cups chicken stock

Arrange the leaves in an ovenproof bowl, place it on a rack in a steamer and steam over gently boiling water for 15 minutes. Meanwhile, blend the cornflour, salt and stock over a gentle heat, bring to the boil and simmer, stirring, until the mixture thickens. Arrange the Chinese leaves on a warmed serving plate, pour over the sauce and serve.

Chinese Leaves with Water Chestnuts

Serves 4

450 g/1 lb Chinese leaves, shredded

45 ml/3 tbsp groundnut (peanut) oil

100 g/4 oz water chestnuts, sliced

250 ml/8 fl oz/1 cup chicken stock

15 ml/1 tbsp soy sauce

15 ml/1 tbsp cornflour (cornstarch)

15 ml/1 tbsp water

Blanch the Chinese leaves in boiling water for 2 minutes then drain. Heat the oil and stir-fry the water chestnuts for 2 minutes. Add the Chinese leaves and stir-fry for 3 minutes. Add the chicken stock and soy sauce, bring to the boil, cover and simmer for 5 minutes. Mix the cornflour and water to a paste, stir into the pan and simmer, stirring, until the sauce clears and thickens.

Courgette Stir-Fry

Serves 4

45 ml/3 tbsp groundnut (peanut) oil
1 spring onion (scallion), chopped
450 g/1 lb courgettes (zucchini), thickly sliced
30 ml/2 tbsp soy sauce
5 ml/1 tsp sugar
120 ml/4 fl oz/½ cup chicken stock
5 ml/1 tsp cornflour (cornstarch)

Heat the oil and fry the spring onion until lightly browned. Add the courgettes and stir-fry for 3 minutes. Add the remaining ingredients and stir-fry for 4 minutes.

Courgettes in Black Bean Sauce

Serves 4

30 ml/2 tbsp groundnut (peanut) oil
1 clove garlic, crushed
5 ml/1 tsp salt
15 ml/1 tbsp chilli bean sauce
450 g/1 lb courgettes (zucchini), thickly sliced
30 ml/2 tbsp rice wine or dry sherry
45 ml/3 tbsp water
15 ml/1 tbsp sesame oil

Heat the oil and fry the garlic, salt and chilli bean sauce for a few seconds. Add the courgettes and stir-fry for 3 minutes until lightly browned. Add the remaining ingredients, including sesame oil to taste, and stir-fry for 1 minute.

Stuffed Courgette Bites

Serves 4

4 large courgettes (zucchini)
225 g/8 oz minced (ground) pork
225 g/8 oz crab meat, flaked
2 eggs, beaten
30 ml/2 tbsp soy sauce
30 ml/2 tbsp oyster sauce
pinch of ground ginger
salt and freshly ground pepper
75 ml/5 tbsp cornflour (cornstarch)
50 g/2 oz/½ cup breadcrumbs
oil for deep-frying

Cut the courgettes in half lengthways and remove the seeds and cores with a spoon. Mix the pork, crab meat, eggs, sauces, ginger, salt and pepper. Bind with the cornflour and breadcrumbs. Cover and chill for 30 minutes. Fill the courgettes with the mixture then cut them into chunks. Heat the oil and deep-fry the courgettes until golden. Drain on kitchen paper before serving.

Cucumber with Prawns

Serves 4

45 ml/3 tbsp groundnut (peanut) oil
100 g/4 oz peeled prawns
1 cucumber, peeled and thickly sliced
30 ml/2 tbsp soy sauce
5 ml/1 tsp rice wine or dry sherry
5 ml/1 tsp brown sugar
salt
45 ml/3 tbsp water

Heat the oil and stir-fry the prawns for 30 seconds. Add the cucumber and stir-fry for 1 minute. Add the soy sauce, wine or sherry and sugar and season with salt. Stir-fry for 3 minutes, adding a little water if necessary. Serve immediately.

Cucumbers with Sesame Oil

Serves 4

1 large cucumber

salt

30 ml/2 tbsp sesame oil

2.5 ml/½ tsp sugar

Peel the cucumber and cut in half lengthways. Scoop out the seeds then cut into thick slices. Arrange the cucumber slices in a colander and sprinkle generously with salt. Leave to stand for 1 hour then press out as much moisture as possible. Heat the oil and stir-fry the cucumbers for 2 minutes until softened. Stir in the sugar and serve at once.

Stuffed Cucumbers

Serves 4

225 g/8 oz minced (ground) pork
1 egg, beaten
30 ml/2 tbsp cornflour (cornstarch)
15 ml/1 tbsp rice wine or dry sherry
30 ml/2 tbsp soy sauce
salt and freshly ground pepper
2 large cucumbers
30 ml/2 tbsp plain (all-purpose) flour
45 ml/3 tbsp groundnut (peanut) oil
150 ml/¼ pt/generous ½ cup chicken stock
30 ml/2 tbsp water

Mix together the pork, egg, half the cornflour, the wine or sherry and half the soy sauce and season with salt and pepper. Peel the cucumbers then cut into 5 cm/2 in chunks. Scoop out some of the seeds to make hollows and fill with stuffing, pressing it down. Dust with flour. Heat the oil and fry the cucumber pieces, stuffing side down, until lightly browned. Turn over and cook until the other side is browned. Add the stock and soy sauce, bring to the boil, cover and simmer for 20 minutes until tender, turning occasionally. Transfer the cucumbers to a warmed serving plate. Mix the remaining cornflour with the water, stir it into the pan and simmer, stirring, until the sauce clears and thickens. Pour over the cucumbers and serve.

Stir-Fried Dandelion Leaves

Serves 4

30 ml/2 tbsp groundnut (peanut) oil
450 g/1 lb dandelion leaves
5 ml/1 tsp salt
15 ml/1 tbsp sugar

Heat the oil, add the dandelion leaves, salt and sugar and stir-fry over a moderate heat for 5 minutes. Serve at once.

Braised Lettuce

Serves 4

1 head crisp lettuce

15 ml/1 tbsp groundnut (peanut) oil

2.5 ml/½ tsp salt

1 clove garlic, crushed

60 ml/4 tbsp chicken stock

5 ml/1 tsp soy sauce

Separate the lettuce into leaves. Heat the oil and fry the salt and garlic until lightly browned. Add the lettuce and simmer for 1 minute, stirring to coat the lettuce in oil. Add the stock and simmer for 2 minutes. Serve sprinkled with soy sauce.

Stir-Fried Lettuce with Ginger

Serves 4

45 ml/3 tbsp groundnut (peanut) oil
2 cloves garlic, crushed
1 cm/½ in slice ginger root, finely chopped
1 head lettuce, shredded

Heat the oil and fry the garlic and ginger until light golden. Add the lettuce and stir-fry for about 2 minutes until glossy and slightly wilted. Serve at once.

Mangetout with Bamboo Shoots

Serves 4

30 ml/2 tbsp groundnut (peanut) oil
100 g/4 oz minced (ground) pork
100 g/4 oz mushrooms
225 g/8 oz bamboo shoots, sliced
225 g/8 oz mangetout (snow peas)
15 ml/1 tbsp soy sauce
15 ml/1 tbsp cornflour (cornstarch)
5 ml/1 tsp sugar
120 ml/4 fl oz/½ cup chicken stock

Heat the oil and fry the pork until lightly browned. Stir in the mushrooms and bamboo shoots and stir-fry for 2 minutes. Add the mangetout and stir-fry for 2 minutes. Sprinkle with soy sauce. Mix the cornflour, sugar and stock to a paste, stir into the pan and simmer, stirring, until the sauce thickens.

Mangetout with Mushrooms and Ginger

Serves 4

45 ml/3 tbsp groundnut (peanut) oil

3 spring onions (scallions), sliced

1 slice ginger root, minced

225 g/8 oz mushrooms, halved

300 ml/½ pt/1¼ cup chicken stock

10 ml/2 tsp cornflour (cornstarch)

15 ml/1 tbsp water

15 ml/1 tbsp oyster sauce

225 g/8 oz mangetout (snow peas)

Heat the oil and fry the spring onions and ginger until lightly browned. Add the mushrooms and stir-fry for 3 minutes. Add the stock, bring to the boil, cover and simmer for 3 minutes. Blend the cornflour to a paste with the water and oyster sauce, stir it into the pan and simmer, stirring, until the sauce thickens. Stir in the mangetout and heat through before serving.

Chinese Marrow

Serves 4

60 ml/4 tbsp groundnut (peanut) oil
450 g/1 lb marrow, thinly sliced
30 ml/2 tbsp soy sauce
10 ml/2 tsp salt
freshly ground pepper

Heat the oil and stir-fry the marrow slices for 2 minutes. Add the soy sauce, salt and a pinch of pepper and stir-fry for a further 4 minutes.

Stuffed Marrow

Serves 4

450 g/1 lb fish fillets, flaked

5 ml/1 tsp salt

2 spring onions (scallions), chopped

100 g/4 oz smoked ham, chopped

50 g/2 oz/½ cup chopped almonds

1 marrow, halved

oil for deep-frying

250 ml/8 fl oz/1 cup chicken stock

30 ml/2 tbsp cornflour (cornstarch)

15 ml/1 tbsp soy sauce

5 ml/1 tsp sugar

60 ml/4 tbsp water

5 ml/1 tsp sesame oil

15 ml/1 tbsp chopped flat-leaved parsley

Mix the fish, salt, spring onions, ham and almonds. Scoop out the seeds of the marrow and some of the flesh to make a hollow. Press the fish mixture into the marrow. Heat the oil and deep-fry the marrow halves, one at a time if necessary, until golden brown. Transfer to a clean pan and add the stock. Bring to the boil, cover and simmer for 40 minutes. Blend the cornflour, soy sauce, sugar, water and sesame oil to a paste, stir into the pan and simmer, stirring, until the sauce clears and thickens. Serve garnished with parsley.

Mushrooms with Anchovy Sauce

Serves 4

15 ml/1 tbsp groundnut (peanut) oil
450 g/1 lb button mushrooms
2 shallots, sliced
1 stick lemon grass, chopped
1 large tomato, diced
60 ml/4 tbsp chopped flat-leaved parsley
20 ml/4 tsp anchovy paste
50 g/2 oz/½ cup butter
salt and freshly ground pepper
4 slices bread
8 anchovy fillets

Heat the oil and fry the mushrooms, shallots and lemon grass until lightly browned. Add the tomato and half the parsley and stir well. Mix in the anchovy paste and the butter, cut into flakes. Season with salt and pepper. Toast the bread then sprinkle with the remaining parsley. Arrange the anchovy fillets on top and serve with the mushrooms.

Mushrooms and Bamboo Shoots

Serves 4

45 ml/3 tbsp groundnut (peanut) oil
5 ml/1 tsp salt
1 clove garlic, crushed
225 g/8 oz bamboo shoots, sliced
225 g/8 oz mushrooms, sliced
45 ml/3 tbsp soy sauce
15 ml/1 tbsp rice wine or dry sherry
15 ml/1 tbsp sugar
15 ml/1 tbsp cornflour (cornstarch)
90 ml/6 tbsp chicken stock

Heat the oil and fry the salt and garlic until the garlic turns light golden. Add the bamboo shoots and mushrooms and stir-fry for 3 minutes. Add the soy sauce, wine or sherry and sugar and stir-fry for 3 minutes. Mix the cornflour and stock and stir it into the pan. Bring to the boil, stirring, then simmer for a few minutes until the sauce thickens and clears.

Mushrooms with Bamboo Shoots and Mangetout

Serves 4

8 dried Chinese mushrooms
30 ml/2 tbsp groundnut (peanut) oil
100 g/4 oz mangetout (snow peas)
100 g/4 oz bamboo shoots, sliced
60 ml/4 tbsp stock
30 ml/2 tbsp soy sauce
5 ml/1 tsp sugar

Soak the mushrooms in warm water for 30 minutes then drain. Discard the stalks and slice the caps. Heat the oil and fry the mangetout for about 30 seconds then remove from the pan. Add the mushrooms and bamboo shoots and stir-fry until well coated with oil. Add the stock, soy sauce and sugar, bring to the boil, cover and simmer gently for 3 minutes. Return the mangetout to the pan and simmer, uncovered, until heated through. Serve at once.

Mushrooms with Mangetout

Serves 4

30 ml/2 tbsp groundnut (peanut) oil

225 g/8 oz button mushrooms

450 g/1 lb mangetout (snow peas)

15 ml/1 tbsp soy sauce

10 ml/2 tsp sesame oil

5 ml/1 tsp brown sugar

Heat the oil and fry the mushrooms for 5 minutes. Add the mangetout and stir-fry for 1 minute. Add the remaining ingredients and stir-fry for 4 minutes.

Spicy Mushrooms

Serves 4

15 ml/1 tbsp groundnut (peanut) oil
1 clove garlic, finely chopped
1 slice ginger root, minced
2 spring onions (scallions), chopped
225 g/8 oz button mushrooms
15 ml/1 tbsp hoisin sauce
15 ml/1 tbsp rice wine or dry sherry
45 ml/3 tbsp chicken stock
5 ml/1 tsp sesame oil

Heat the oil and stir-fry the garlic, ginger and spring onions for 2 minutes. Add the mushrooms and stir-fry for 2 minutes. Add the remaining ingredients and stir-fry for 5 minutes.

Steamed Mushrooms

Serves 4

18 dried Chinese mushrooms
450 ml/¾ pt/2 cups stock
30 ml/2 tbsp groundnut (peanut) oil
5 ml/1 tsp sugar

Soak the mushrooms in warm water for 30 minutes then drain, reserving 250 ml/8 fl oz/1 cup of soaking liquid. Discard the stalks and arrange the caps in a heatproof bowl. Add the remaining ingredients, stand the bowl on a rack in a steamer, cover and steam over boiling water for about 1 hour.

Steamed Stuffed Mushrooms

Serves 4

450 g/1 lb large mushrooms

225 g/8 oz minced (ground) pork

225 g/8 oz peeled prawns, finely chopped

4 water chestnuts, finely chopped

15 ml/1 tbsp cornflour (cornstarch)

5 ml/1 tsp salt

5 ml/1 tsp sugar

30 ml/2 tbsp soy sauce

120 ml/4 fl oz/½ cup

Remove the stalks from the mushrooms. Chop the stalks and mix them with the remaining ingredients. Arrange the mushroom caps on an ovenproof plate and top with the stuffing mixture, pressing it down into a dome shape. Spoon a little stock over each one, reserving a little stock. Place the plate on a rack in a steamer, cover and steam over gently simmering water for about 45 minutes until the mushrooms are cooked, basting with a little more stock during cooking if necessary.

Straw Mushrooms in Oyster Sauce

Serves 4

15 ml/1 tbsp groundnut (peanut) oil
225 g/8 oz straw mushrooms
120 ml/4 fl oz/½ cup chicken stock
2.5 ml/½ tsp sugar
5 ml/1 tsp oyster sauce
5 ml/1 tsp cornflour (cornstarch)
15 ml/1 tbsp water

Heat the oil and fry the mushrooms gently until well coated. Add the stock, sugar and oyster sauce, bring to the boil then simmer gently until the mushrooms are tender. Mix the cornflour and water to a paste, stir into the pan and simmer, stirring, until the sauce clears and thickens.

Baked Onions

Serves 4

8 large onions
salt and freshly ground pepper
30 ml/2 tbsp groundnut (peanut) oil
120 ml/4 fl oz/½ cup water
15 ml/1 tbsp cornflour (cornstarch)
15 ml/1 tbsp chopped fresh parsley

Put the onions in a pan and just cover with boiling salted water. Cover and simmer for 5 minutes then drain. Arrange the onions in an ovenproof dish, season with salt and pepper and brush with oil. Pour in the water, cover and bake in a preheated oven at 190°C/375°F/gas mark 5 for 1 hour. Blend the cornflour with a little water and stir it into the onion liquid. Bake for a further 5 minutes, stirring occasionally, until the sauce thickens. Serve garnished with parsley.

Curried Onions with Peas

Serves 4

450 g/1 lb pearl onions

10 ml/2 tsp salt

225 g/8 oz peas

45 ml/3 tbsp groundnut (peanut) oil

10 ml/2 tsp curry powder

freshly ground pepper

Place the onions in a pan and just cover with boiling water. Season with 5 ml/1 tsp of salt and boil for 5 minutes. Cover and boil for a further 10 minutes. Add the peas and cook for a further 5 minutes then drain. Heat the oil and fry the curry powder, remaining salt and remaining pepper for 30 seconds. Add the drained vegetables and stir-fry until hot and glazed with the curry oil.

Pearl Onions in Orange-Ginger Sauce

Serves 4

3 oranges

2 red chilli peppers

15 ml/1 tbsp walnut oil

450 g/1 lb pearl onions

1 slice ginger root, chopped

10 ml/2 tsp sugar

10 ml/2 tsp cider vinegar

15 ml/1 tbsp red peppercorns

salt

5 ml/1 tsp grated lemon rind

a few coriander leaves

Using a zester, cut the orange peel into narrow slivers. Halve the oranges and squeeze the juice. Halve the chilli peppers and remove the seeds. Heat the oil and stir-fry the onions, ginger and chilli peppers for 1 minute. Add the sugar then simmer until the onions are translucent. Mix in the orange juice, cider vinegar, peppercorns and orange rind and season with salt. Stir in the lemon rind and most of the coriander leaves. Arrange on a warmed serving plate and garnish with the remaining coriander leaves.

Onion Custard

Serves 4

4 rashers bacon
450 g/1 lb onions, sliced
50 g/2 oz/½ cup cornflour (cornstarch)
2 eggs, lightly beaten
120 ml/4 fl oz/½ cup water
pinch of grated nutmeg
10 ml/2 tsp salt

Fry the bacon until crisp then drain and chop. Add the onions to the pan and fry until softened. Beat the cornflour with the eggs and water and season with nutmeg and salt. Mix the bacon with the onions and place in a greased ovenproof dish. Top with the egg mixture and stand the dish in a roasting tin half filled with water. Bake in a preheated oven at 180°C/ 350°F/gas mark 4 for 45 minutes until the custard is set.

Pak Choi

Serves 4

45 ml/3 tbsp groundnut (peanut) oil
2 spring onions (scallions), chopped
450 g/1 lb pak choi, shredded
15 ml/1 tbsp soy sauce
2.5 ml/½ tsp sugar
120 ml/4 fl oz/½ cup chicken stock
5 ml/1 tsp cornflour (cornstarch)

Heat the oil and fry the spring onions until lightly browned. Add the pak choi and stir-fry for 3 minutes. Add the remaining ingredients and stir-fry for 2 minutes.

Peas with Mushrooms

Serves 4

45 ml/3 tbsp groundnut (peanut) oil

1 spring onion (scallion), chopped

225 g/8 oz mushrooms, halved

225 g/8 oz frozen peas

30 ml/2 tbsp soy sauce

5 ml/1 tsp sugar

120 ml/4 fl oz/½ cup chicken stock

5 ml/1 tsp cornflour (cornstarch)

Heat the oil and fry the spring onion until lightly browned. Add the mushrooms and stir-fry for 3 minutes. Add the peas and stir-fry for 4 minutes. Add the remaining ingredients and stir-fry for 2 minutes.

Stir-Fried Peppers

Serves 4

30 ml/2 tbsp groundnut (peanut) oil
2 green peppers, cubed
2 red peppers, cubed
15 ml/1 tbsp chicken stock or water
5 ml/1 tsp salt
5 ml/1 tsp brown sugar

Heat the oil until very hot, add the peppers and stir-fry until the skins wrinkle slightly. Add the stock or water, salt and sugar and stir-fry for 2 minutes.

Pepper and Bean Stir-Fry

Serves 4

30 ml/2 tbsp groundnut (peanut) oil
2 cloves garlic, crushed
5 ml/1 tsp salt
2 red peppers, cut into strips
225 g/8 oz French beans
5 ml/1 tsp sugar
30 ml/2 tbsp water

Heat the oil and stir-fry the garlic, salt, peppers and beans for 3 minutes. Add the sugar and water and stir-fry for about 5 minutes until the vegetables are tender but still crisp.

Fish-Stuffed Peppers

Serves 4

225 g/8 oz fish fillets, flaked
2 spring onions (scallions), minced
30 ml/2 tbsp cornflour (cornstarch)
15 ml/1 tbsp groundnut (peanut) oil
30 ml/2 tbsp water
salt and freshly ground pepper
4 green peppers
120 ml/4 fl oz/½ cup chicken stock
2.5 ml/½ tsp salt
60 ml/4 tbsp water

Mix together the fish, spring onions, half the cornflour, the oil and water and season with salt and pepper. Cut the tops off the peppers and scoop out the seeds. Fill with the stuffing mixture and replace the tops as lids. Stand the peppers upright in a pan and add the stock. Bring to the boil and season with salt and pepper. Cover and simmer for 1 hour. Transfer the peppers to a warmed serving dish. Blend the remaining cornflour and water to a paste, stir into the pan and bring to the boil. Simmer, stirring, until the sauce clears and thickens. Pour over the peppers and serve at once.

Pork-Stuffed Peppers

Serves 4

30 ml/2 tbsp groundnut (peanut) oil

225 g/8 oz minced (ground) pork

2 spring onions (scallions), chopped

4 water chestnuts, chopped

30 ml/2 tbsp soy sauce

salt and freshly ground pepper

4 green peppers

120 ml/4 fl oz/½ cup chicken stock

2.5 ml/½ tsp salt

15 ml/1 tbsp cornflour (cornstarch)

60 ml/4 tbsp water

Heat the oil and fry the pork, spring onions and water chestnuts until lightly browned. Remove from the heat, stir half the soy sauce and season with salt and pepper. Cut the tops off the peppers and scoop out the seeds. Fill with the stuffing mixture and replace the tops as lids. Stand the peppers upright in a pan and add the stock. Bring to the boil and season with salt and pepper. Cover and simmer for 1 hour. Transfer the peppers to a warmed serving dish. Blend the cornflour, remaining soy sauce and water to a paste, stir into the pan and bring to the boil.

Simmer, stirring, until the sauce clears and thickens. Pour over the peppers and serve at once.

Vegetable-Stuffed Peppers

Serves 4

30 ml/2 tbsp groundnut (peanut) oil

2 carrots, grated

1 onion, grated

45 ml/3 tbsp tomato ketchup (catsup)

5 ml/1 tsp sugar

salt and freshly ground pepper

4 green peppers

120 ml/4 fl oz/½ cup chicken stock

2.5 ml/½ tsp salt

15 ml/1 tbsp cornflour (cornstarch)

15 ml/1 tbsp soy sauce

60 ml/4 tbsp water

Heat the oil and fry the carrots and onions until slightly softened. Remove from the heat and stir in the tomato ketchup and sugar. Season with salt and pepper. Cut the tops off the peppers and scoop out the seeds. Fill with the stuffing mixture and replace the tops as lids. Stand the peppers upright in a pan and add the stock. Bring to the boil and season with salt and pepper. Cover and simmer for 1 hour. Transfer the peppers to a warmed serving dish. Blend the cornflour, soy sauce and water to a paste, stir into the pan and bring to the boil. Simmer, stirring, until the sauce clears and thickens. Pour over the peppers and serve at once.

Deep-Fried Potatoes and Carrots

Serves 4

2 carrots, diced
450 g/1 lb potatoes
15 ml/1 tbsp cornflour (cornstarch)
oil for deep-frying
30 ml/2 tbsp groundnut (peanut) oil
5 ml/1 tsp salt
15 ml/1 tbsp rice wine or dry sherry
120 ml/4 fl oz/½ cup chicken stock
5 ml/1 tsp sugar
5 ml/1 tsp soy sauce

Blanch the carrots in boiling water for 3 minutes then drain. Cut the potatoes into chips and dust with a little cornflour. Heat the oil and deep-fry until crisp then drain. Heat the oil and salt and stir-fry the carrots until coated with oil. Add the wine or sherry and stock, bring to the boil, cover and simmer for 2 minutes. Blend the remaining cornflour to a paste with the sugar and soy sauce. Stir into the pan and simmer, stirring, until the sauce thickens. Add the potatoes and reheat. Serve at once.

Potato Sauté

Serves 4

350 g/12 oz potatoes, peeled and cut into matchsticks

30 ml/2 tbsp groundnut (peanut) oil

1 clove garlic, crushed

3 spring onions (scallions), chopped

15 ml/1 tbsp soy sauce

5 ml/1 tsp wine vinegar

salt and freshly ground pepper

Blanch the potatoes in boiling water for 20 seconds then drain. Heat the oil and fry the garlic and spring onions until lightly browned. Add the potatoes and stir-fry for 2 minutes. Add the soy sauce and wine vinegar and season to taste with salt and pepper. Fry for a few minutes until the potatoes are cooked and lightly browned.

Spiced Potatoes

Serves 4

30 ml/2 tbsp groundnut (peanut) oil
350 g/12 oz potatoes, peeled and diced
1 clove garlic, crushed
2.5 ml/½ tsp salt
2 spring onions (scallions), chopped
2 dried chilli peppers, seeded and chopped

Heat the oil and fry the potatoes until lightly golden. Remove them from the pan. Reheat the oil and fry the garlic, salt, spring onions and chilli peppers until lightly browned. Return the potatoes to the pan and stir-fry until the potatoes are cooked.

Pumpkin with Rice Noodles

Serves 4

350 g/12 oz rice noodles
15 ml/1 tbsp groundnut (peanut) oil
2 spring onions (scallions), sliced
225 g/8 oz pumpkin, cubed
250 ml/8 fl oz/1 cup chicken stock
2.5 ml/½ tsp sugar
salt and freshly ground pepper
100 g/4 oz peeled prawns

Blanch the noodles in boiling water for 2 minutes then drain. Heat the oil and stir-fry the spring onions for 30 seconds. Add the pumpkin and stir-fry for 1 minute. Add the stock and noodles, bring to the boil and simmer, uncovered, for about 5 minutes until the pumpkin is almost cooked. Add the sugar and season with salt and pepper. Simmer for about 10 minutes until the noodles are just tender and the liquid has reduced slightly. Add the prawns and heat through before serving.

Shallots in Malt Beer

Serves 4

15 ml/1 tbsp walnut oil
450 g/1 lb shallots
10 ml/2 tsp brown sugar
5 ml/1 tsp red peppercorns
250 ml/8 fl oz/1 cup malt beer
45 ml/3 tbsp balsamic vinegar
salt and freshly ground pepper
2.5 ml/½ tsp paprika
1 lamb's lettuce

Heat the oil and fry the shallots until golden brown. Add the sugar and stir-fry until translucent. Add the peppercorns, beer and balsamic vinegar and simmer for 1 minute. Season with salt, pepper and paprika. Arrange the lettuce leaves around the edge of a warmed serving plate and spoon the shallots into the centre.

Spinach with Garlic

Serves 4

30 ml/2 tbsp groundnut (peanut) oil

450 g/1 lb spinach leaves

2.5 ml/½ tsp salt

3 cloves garlic, crushed

15 ml/1 tbsp soy sauce

Heat the oil, add the spinach and salt and stir-fry for 3 minutes until the spinach begins to wilt. Add the garlic and soy sauce and stir-fry for 3 minutes before serving.

Spinach with Mushrooms

Serves 4–6

8 dried Chinese mushrooms
75 ml/5 tbsp groundnut (peanut) oil
60 ml/4 tbsp soy sauce
15 ml/1 tbsp rice wine or dry sherry
5 ml/1 tsp sugar
salt
15 ml/1 tbsp cornflour (cornstarch)
15 ml/1 tbsp water
450 g/1 lb spinach

Soak the mushrooms in warm water for 30 minutes then drain, reserving 120 ml/4 fl oz/½ cup of soaking liquid. Discard the stalks and cut the caps in half, if large. Heat half the oil and fry the mushrooms for 2 minutes. Stir in the soy sauce, wine or sherry, sugar and a pinch of salt and mix well. Add the mushroom liquid, bring to the boil, cover and simmer for 10 minutes. Blend the cornflour and water to a paste, stir it into the sauce and simmer, stirring, until the sauce thickens. Leave over a very low heat to keep warm. Meanwhile, heat the remaining oil in a separate pan, add the spinach and stir-fry for about 2 minutes until softened. Transfer to a warmed serving dish, pour over the mushrooms and serve.

Spinach with Ginger

Serves 4

30 ml/2 tbsp groundnut (peanut) oil
1 slice ginger root, minced
1 clove garlic, crushed
5 ml/1 tsp salt
450 g/1 lb spinach
5 ml/1 tsp sugar
10 ml/2 tsp sesame oil

Heat the oil and stir-fry the ginger, garlic and salt until lightly browned. Add the spinach and stir-fry for 3 minutes until wilted. Add the sugar and sesame oil and stir-fry for 3 minutes. Serve hot or cold.

Spinach with Peanuts

Serves 4

30 ml/2 tbsp peanuts
450 g/1 lb spinach, shredded
2.5 ml/½ tsp salt
100 g/4 oz smoked ham, chopped
15 ml/1 tbsp groundnut (peanut) oil

Toast the peanuts in a dry pan then chop coarsely. Blanch the spinach in boiling water for 2 minutes then drain well and chop. Mix in the peanuts, salt, ham and oil and serve at once.

Vegetable Chow Mein

Serves 4

6 dried Chinese mushrooms

450 g/1 lb spinach

45 ml/3 tbsp groundnut (peanut) oil

100 g/4 oz bamboo shoots, sliced

2.5 ml/½ tsp salt

30 ml/2 tbsp soy sauce

soft-fried noodles

Soak the mushrooms in warm water for 30 minutes then drain. Discard the stalks and slice the caps. Halve the spinach leaves. Heat the oil and stir-fry the mushrooms and bamboo shoots for 4 minutes. Add the spinach, salt and soy sauce and stir-fry for 1 minute. Add the drained noodles and stir gently until heated through.

Mixed Vegetables

Serves 4

2 onions

30 ml/2 tbsp groundnut (peanut) oil

15 ml/1 tbsp grated ginger root

225 g/8 oz broccoli florets

225 g/8 oz spinach, chopped

225 g/8 oz mangetout (snow peas)

4 stalks celery, diagonally sliced

6 spring onions (scallions), diagonally sliced

175 ml/6 fl oz/¾ cup vegetable stock

Cut the onions into wedges and separate the layers. Heat the oil and stir-fry the onions, ginger and broccoli for 1 minute. Add the remaining vegetables and toss lightly. Add the stock and toss until the vegetables are completely coated. Bring to the boil, cover and simmer for 3 minutes until the vegetables are tender but still crisp.

Mixed Vegetables with Ginger

Serves 4

100 g/4 oz cauliflower florets

45 ml/3 tbsp groundnut (peanut) oil

2 slices ginger root, minced

1 spring onion (scallion), chopped

100 g/4 oz bamboo shoots, sliced

100 g/4 oz mushrooms, sliced

100 g/4 oz Chinese cabbage, shredded

30 ml/2 tbsp soy sauce

120 ml/4 fl oz/½ cup chicken stock

salt and freshly ground pepper

Blanch the cauliflower in boiling water for 3 minutes then drain. Heat the oil and stir-fry the ginger for 1 minute. Add the vegetables and stir-fry for 3 minutes until coated with oil. Add the soy sauce and stock and season with salt and pepper. Stir-fry for a further 2 minutes until the vegetables are just tender but still crisp.

Vegetable Spring Rolls

Serves 4

6 dried Chinese mushrooms

30 ml/2 tbsp groundnut (peanut) oil

2.5 ml/½ tsp salt

2 cloves garlic, finely chopped

2 stalks celery, chopped

1 green pepper, sliced

50 g/2 oz bamboo shoots, sliced

100 g/4 oz Chinese leaves, shredded

100 g/4 oz bean sprouts

4 water chestnuts, cut into strips

3 spring onions (scallions), chopped

15 ml/1 tbsp soy sauce

5 ml/1 tsp sugar

8 spring roll skins

groundnut (peanut) oil for frying

Soak the mushrooms in warm water for 30 minutes then drain. Discard the stems and chop the caps. Heat the oil, salt and garlic until the garlic turns golden then add the mushrooms and stir-fry for 2 minutes. Add the celery, pepper and bamboo shoots and stir-fry for 3 minutes. Add the cabbage, bean sprouts, chestnuts and spring onions and stir-fry for 2 minutes. Stir in the soy sauce and sugar, remove from the heat and leave to stand for 2 minutes. Turn into a colander and leave to drain. Place a few spoonfuls of the filling mixture in the centre of each spring roll skin, fold up the bottom, fold in the sides, then roll upwards, enclosing the filling. Seal the edge with a little flour and water mixture then leave to dry for 30 minutes. Heat the oil and fry the spring rolls for about 10 minutes until crisp and golden brown. Drain well before serving.

Simple Stir-Fried Vegetables

Serves 4

45 ml/3 tbsp groundnut (peanut) oil

5 ml/1 tsp salt

2 slices ginger root, minced

450 g/1 lb mixed vegetables such as sliced bamboo shoots, blanched bean sprouts, broccoli florets, sliced carrots, cauliflower florets, diced peppers

120 ml/4 fl oz/½ cup chicken or vegetable stock

15 ml/1 tbsp soy sauce

5 ml/1 tsp sugar

Heat the oil and stir-fry the salt and ginger until lightly browned. Add the vegetables and stir-fry for 3 minutes until well coated with oil. Add the stock, soy sauce and sugar and stir-fry for about 2 minutes until heated through.

Vegetables with Honey

Serves 4

15 ml/1 tbsp groundnut (peanut) oil
1 slice ginger root, chopped
2 cloves garlic, chopped
100 g/4 oz baby sweetcorn
2 spring onions (scallions), sliced
1 red pepper, diced
1 green pepper, diced
100 g/4 oz mushrooms, halved
15 ml/1 tbsp honey
15 ml/1 tbsp fruit vinegar
10 ml/2 tsp soy sauce
salt and freshly ground pepper

Heat the oil and fry the ginger and garlic until lightly browned. Add the vegetables and stir-fry for 1 minute. Add the honey, fruit vinegar and soy sauce and season with salt and pepper. Stir together well and heat through before serving.

Fried Spring Vegetables

Serves 4

45 ml/3 tbsp groundnut (peanut) oil
2 cloves garlic, crushed
salt
30 ml/2 tbsp soy sauce
30 ml/2 tbsp hoisin sauce
6 spring onions (scallions), chopped
1 red pepper, chopped
1 green pepper, chopped
100 g/4 oz bean sprouts
225 g/8 oz mangetout (snow peas), cut into 4
5 ml/1 tsp tomato purée (paste)
5 ml/1 tsp cornflour (cornstarch)
120 ml/4 fl oz/½ cup chicken stock
few drops of lemon juice
60 ml/4 tbsp chopped chives

Heat the oil and fry the garlic and salt until lightly browned. Add the soy and hoisin sauces and stir-fry for 1 minute. Add the peppers, bean sprouts and mangetout and cook, stirring, until they are just tender but still crisp. Stir the tomato purée and cornflour into the stock then add it to the pan. Bring to the boil and simmer, stirring, until the sauce thickens. Sprinkle with lemon juice, stir, then serve sprinkled with chives.

Marinated Steamed Vegetables

Serves 4

30 ml/2 tbsp groundnut (peanut) oil
225 g/8 oz broccoli florets
225 g/8 oz cauliflower florets
100 g/4 oz oyster mushrooms
2 carrots, thinly sliced
1 stick celery, thinly sliced
120 ml/4 fl oz/½ cup dry white wine
30 ml/2 tbsp plum sauce
30 ml/2 tbsp soy sauce
juice of 1 orange
5 ml/1 tsp freshly ground pepper
30 ml/2 tbsp wine vinegar

Heat the oil and stir-fry the vegetables for about 5 minutes then transfer them to a bowl. Add the wine, plum sauce, soy sauce, orange juice and pepper and toss well to mix. Cover and refrigerate overnight.

Place the marinated vegetables in a steamer, cover and cook over gently boiling water to which the wine vinegar has been added for about 15 minutes.

Vegetable Surprises

Serves 4

225 g/8 oz broccoli florets
225 g/8 oz cauliflower florets
225 g/8 oz brussels sprouts
30 ml/2 tbsp honey
30 ml/2 tbsp soy sauce
30 ml/2 tbsp wine vinegar
5 ml/1 tsp five-spice powder
salt and freshly ground pepper
225 g/8 oz/2 cups plain (all-purpose) flour
250 ml/8 fl oz/1 cup dry white wine
2 eggs, separated
15 ml/1 tbsp grated lemon rind
oil for deep-frying

Blanch the vegetables for 1 minute in boiling water then drain. Mix together the honey, soy sauce, wine vinegar, five-spice powder, salt and pepper. Place the vegetables in the marinade, cover and chill for 2 hours, stirring occasionally. Mix the flour, wine and egg yolks until smooth. Whisk the egg whites until stiff then fold them into the batter. Season with salt, pepper and lemon rind. Drain the vegetables and coat them in the batter. Heat the oil and deep-fry until golden brown. Drain on kitchen paper before serving.

Sweet and Sour Mixed Vegetables

Serves 4

45 ml/3 tbsp groundnut (peanut) oil
2.5 ml/½ tsp salt
2 cloves garlic, crushed
2 carrots, sliced
1 green pepper, cubed
100 g/4 oz bamboo shoots, cut into strips
1 onion, cut into wedges
100 g/4 oz water chestnuts, cut into strips
100 g/4 oz/½ cup sugar
60 ml/4 tbsp chicken stock
60 ml/4 tbsp wine vinegar
30 ml/2 tbsp soy sauce
15 ml/1 tbsp cornflour (cornstarch)

Heat the oil, salt and garlic until the garlic turns light golden. Add the carrots, pepper, bamboo shoots and onions and stir-fry for 3 minutes. Add the water chestnuts and stir-fry for 2 minutes. Mix together the sugar, stock, wine vinegar, soy sauce and cornflour then stir it into the pan. Cook, stirring, until the sauce thickens and clears.

Vegetables in Tomato Sauce

Serves 4

30 ml/2 tbsp groundnut (peanut) oil
2 cloves garlic, crushed
5 ml/1 tsp salt
100 g/4 oz smoked bacon, diced
30 ml/2 tbsp tomato purée (paste)
30 ml/2 tbsp soy sauce
30 ml/2 tbsp honey
30 ml/2 tbsp hoisin sauce
300 ml/½ pt/1¼ cups vegetable stock
1 red pepper, cut into strips
1 green pepper, cut into strips
1 stick celery, cut into strips
100 g/4 oz bean sprouts
100 g/4 oz green peas
10 ml/2 tsp wine vinegar

Heat the oil and fry the garlic and salt until lightly browned. Add the bacon and fry until crisp. Blend together the tomato purée, soy sauce, honey, hoisin sauce and stock. Add the vegetables to the pan and stir-fry for 2 minutes until coated in oil. Add the stock mixture, bring to the boil, cover and simmer for about 20 minutes until cooked.

Water Chestnut Cakes

Serves 4

100 g/4 oz sesame seeds
900 g/2 lb water chestnuts
15 ml/1 tbsp plain (all-purpose) flour
5 ml/1 tsp salt
freshly ground pepper
225 g/8 oz red bean paste
oil for deep-frying
120 ml/4 fl oz/½ cup vegetable stock
15 ml/1 tbsp sesame oil
5 ml/1 tsp cinnamon

Toast the sesame seeds in a dry pan until lightly browned. Mince the water chestnuts and drain off a little of the water. Mix with the flour, salt and pepper and shape into small balls. Press a little bean paste into the centre of each one. Coat the cakes in sesame seeds. Heat the oil and deep-fry the cakes for about 3 minutes then remove from the pan and drain. Pour off all but 30 ml/2 tbsp of oil from the pan then return the cakes to the pan and fry over a low heat for 4 minutes. Add the remaining ingredients, bring to a simmer and simmer until most of the liquid has been absorbed. Transfer to a warmed serving plate and serve at once.

Simple Chicken Stir-Fry

Serves 4

1 chicken breast, thinly sliced
2 slices ginger root, minced
2 spring onions (scallions), minced
15 ml/1 tbsp cornflour (cornstarch)
15 ml/1 tbsp rice wine or dry sherry
30 ml/2 tbsp water
2.5 ml/½ tsp salt
45 ml/3 tbsp groundnut (peanut) oil
100 g/4 oz bamboo shoots, sliced
100 g/4 oz mushrooms, sliced
100 g/4 oz bean sprouts
15 ml/1 tbsp soy sauce
5 ml/1 tsp sugar
120 ml/4 fl oz/½ cup chicken stock

Place the chicken in a bowl. Mix the ginger, spring onions, cornflour, wine or sherry, water and salt, stir into the chicken and leave to stand for 1 hour. Heat half the oil and stir-fry the chicken until lightly browned then remove it from the pan. Heat the remaining oil and stir-fry the bamboo shoots, mushrooms and bean sprouts for 4 minutes. Add the soy sauce, sugar and stock, bring to the boil, cover and simmer for 5 minutes until the vegetables are just tender. Return the chicken to the pan, stir well and reheat gently before serving.

Chicken in Tomato Sauce

Serves 4

30 ml/2 tbsp groundnut (peanut) oil
5 ml/1 tsp salt
2 cloves garlic, crushed
450 g/1 lb chicken, cubed
300 ml/½ pt/1¼ cups chicken stock
120 ml/4 fl oz/½ cup tomato ketchup (catsup)
15 ml/1 tbsp cornflour (cornstarch)
4 spring onions (scallions), sliced

Heat the oil with the salt and garlic until the garlic is lightly golden. Add the chicken and stir-fry until lightly browned. Add most of the stock, bring to the boil, cover and simmer for about 15 minutes until the chicken is tender. Stir the remaining stock with the ketchup and cornflour and stir it into the pan. Simmer, stirring, until the sauce thickens and clears. If the sauce is too thin, leave it simmering for a while until it has reduced. Add the spring onions and simmer for 2 minutes before serving.

Chicken with Tomatoes

Serves 4

225 g/8 oz chicken, diced

15 ml/1 tbsp cornflour (cornstarch)

15 ml/1 tbsp soy sauce

15 ml/1 tbsp rice wine or dry sherry

45 ml/3 tbsp groundnut (peanut) oil

1 onion, diced

60 ml/4 tbsp chicken stock

5 ml/1 tsp salt

5 ml/1 tsp sugar

2 tomatoes, skinned and diced

Mix the chicken with the cornflour, soy sauce and wine or sherry and leave to stand for 30 minutes. Heat the oil and fry the chicken until lightly coloured. Add the onion and stir-fry until softened. Add the stock, salt and sugar, bring to the boil and stir gently over a low heat until the chicken is cooked. Add the tomatoes and stir until heated through.

Poached Chicken with Tomatoes

Serves 4

4 chicken portions

4 tomatoes, skinned and quartered

15 ml/1 tbsp rice wine or dry sherry

15 ml/1 tbsp groundnut (peanut) oil

salt

Place the chicken in a pan and just cover with cold water. Bring to the boil, cover and simmer for 20 minutes. Add the tomatoes, wine or sherry, oil and salt, cover and simmer for a further 10 minutes until the chicken is cooked. Arrange the chicken on a warmed serving plate and chop into serving pieces. Reheat the sauce and pour over the chicken to serve.

Chicken and Tomatoes with Black Bean Sauce

Serves 4

45 ml/3 tbsp groundnut (peanut) oil
1 clove garlic, crushed
45 ml/3 tbsp black bean sauce
225 g/8 oz chicken, diced
15 ml/1 tbsp rice wine or dry sherry
5 ml/1 tsp sugar
15 ml/1 tbsp soy sauce
90 ml/6 tbsp chicken stock
3 tomatoes, skinned and quartered
10 ml/2 tsp cornflour (cornstarch)
45 ml/3 tbsp water

Heat the oil and fry the garlic for 30 seconds. Add the black bean sauce and fry for 30 seconds then add the chicken and stir until well coated in oil. Add the wine or sherry, sugar, soy sauce and stock, bring to the boil, cover and simmer for about 5 minutes until the chicken is cooked. Mix the cornflour and water to a paste, stir it into the pan and simmer, stirring, until the sauce clears and thickens.

Quick-Cooked Chicken with Vegetables

Serves 4

1 egg white

50 g/2 oz cornflour (cornstarch)

225 g/8 oz chicken breasts, cut into strips

75 ml/5 tbsp groundnut (peanut) oil

200 g/7 oz bamboo shoots, cut into strips

50 g/2 oz bean sprouts

1 green pepper, cut into strips

3 spring onions (scallions), sliced

1 slice ginger root, minced

1 clove garlic, minced

15 ml/1 tbsp rice wine or dry sherry

Beat the egg white and cornflour then dip the chicken strips in the mixture. Heat the oil to moderately hot and fry the chicken for a few minutes until just cooked. Remove from the pan and drain well. Add the bamboo shoots, bean sprouts, pepper, onions, ginger and garlic to the pan and stir-fry for 3 minutes. Add the wine or sherry and return the chicken to the pan. Stir together well and heat through before serving.

Walnut Chicken

Serves 4

45 ml/3 tbsp groundnut (peanut) oil

2 spring onions (scallions), chopped

1 slice ginger root, minced

450 g/1 lb chicken breast, very thinly sliced

50 g/2 oz ham, shredded

30 ml/2 tbsp soy sauce

30 ml/2 tbsp rice wine or dry sherry

5 ml/1 tsp sugar

5 ml/1 tsp salt

100 g/4 oz/1 cup walnuts, chopped

Heat the oil and stir-fry the onions and ginger for 1 minute. Add the chicken and ham and stir-fry for 5 minutes until almost cooked. Add the soy sauce, wine or sherry, sugar and salt and stir-fry for 3 minutes. Add the walnuts and stir-fry for 1 minute until the ingredients are thoroughly blended.

Chicken with Walnuts

Serves 4

100 g/4 oz/1 cup shelled walnuts, halved
oil for deep-frying
45 ml/3 tbsp groundnut (peanut) oil
2 slices ginger root, minced
225 g/8 oz chicken, diced
100 g/4 oz bamboo shoots, sliced
75 ml/5 tbsp chicken stock

Prepare the walnuts, heat the oil and deep-fry the walnuts until golden brown then drain well. Heat the groundnut oil and fry the ginger for 30 seconds. Add the chicken and stir-fry until lightly browned. Add the remaining ingredients, bring to the boil and simmer, stirring, until the chicken is cooked.

Chicken with Water Chestnuts

Serves 4

45 ml/3 tbsp groundnut (peanut) oil

2 cloves garlic, crushed

2 spring onions (scallions), chopped

1 slice ginger root, chopped

225 g/8 oz chicken breast, cut into slivers

100 g/4 oz water chestnuts, cut into slivers

45 ml/3 tbsp soy sauce

15 ml/1 tbsp rice wine or dry sherry

5 ml/1 tsp cornflour (cornstarch)

Heat the oil and fry the garlic, spring onions and ginger until lightly browned. Add the chicken and stir-fry for 5 minutes. Add the water chestnuts and stir-fry for 3 minutes. Add the soy sauce, wine or sherry and cornflour and stir-fry for about 5 minutes until the chicken is cooked through.

Savoury Chicken with Water Chestnuts

Serves 4

30 ml/2 tbsp groundnut (peanut) oil

4 chicken pieces

3 spring onions (scallions), chopped

2 cloves garlic, crushed

1 slice ginger root, chopped

250 ml/8 fl oz/1 cup soy sauce

30 ml/2 tbsp rice wine or dry sherry

30 ml/2 tbsp brown sugar

5 ml/1 tsp salt

375 ml/13 fl oz/1¼ cups water

225 g/8 oz water chestnuts, sliced

15 ml/1 tbsp cornflour (cornstarch)

Heat the oil and fry the chicken pieces until golden brown. Add the spring onions, garlic and ginger and fry for 2 minutes. Add the soy sauce, wine or sherry, sugar and salt and stir together well. Add the water and bring to the boil, cover and simmer for 20 minutes. Add the water chestnuts, cover and cook for a further 20 minutes. Mix the cornflour with a little water, stir it into the sauce and simmer, stirring, until the sauce clears and thickens.

Chicken Wontons

Serves 4

4 dried Chinese mushrooms
450 g/1 lb chicken breast, shredded
225 g/8 oz mixed vegetables, chopped
1 spring onion (scallion), chopped
15 ml/1 tbsp soy sauce
2.5 ml/½ tsp salt
40 wonton skins
1 egg, beaten

Soak the mushrooms in warm water for 30 minutes then drain. Discard the stalks and chop the caps. Mix with the chicken, vegetables, soy sauce and salt.

To fold the wontons, hold the skin in the palm of your left hand and spoon a little filling into the centre. Moisten the edges with egg and fold the skin into a triangle, sealing the edges. Moisten the corners with egg and twist them together.

Bring a saucepan of water to the boil. Drop in the wontons and simmer for about 10 minutes until they float to the top.

Crispy Chicken Wings

Serves 4

900 g/2 lb chicken wings
60 ml/4 tbsp rice wine or dry sherry
60 ml/4 tbsp soy sauce
50 g/2 oz/½ cup cornflour (cornstarch)
groundnut (peanut) oil for deep-frying

Place the chicken wings in a bowl. Mix together the remaining ingredients and pour over the chicken wings, stirring well so that they are coated in the sauce. Cover and leave to stand for 30 minutes. Heat the oil and deep-fry the chicken a few at a time until cooked through and dark brown. Drain well on kitchen paper and keep warm while you fry the remaining chicken.

Five-Spice Chicken Wings

Serves 4

30 ml/2 tbsp groundnut (peanut) oil

2 cloves garlic, crushed

450 g/1 lb chicken wings

250 ml/8 fl oz/1 cup chicken stock

30 ml/2 tbsp soy sauce

5 ml/1 tsp sugar

5 ml/1 tsp five-spice powder

Heat the oil and garlic until the garlic is lightly browned. Add the chicken and fry until lightly browned. Add the remaining ingredients, stirring well, and bring to the boil. Cover and simmer for about 15 minutes until the chicken is cooked through. Remove the lid and continue to simmer, stirring occasionally, until almost all the liquid has evaporated. Serve hot or cold.

Marinated Chicken Wings

Serves 4

45 ml/3 tbsp soy sauce

45 ml/3 tbsp rice wine or dry sherry

30 ml/2 tbsp brown sugar

5 ml/1 tsp grated ginger root

2 cloves garlic, crushed

6 spring onions (scallions), sliced

450 g/1 lb chicken wings

30 ml/2 tbsp groundnut (peanut) oil

225 g/8 oz bamboo shoots, sliced

20 ml/4 tsp cornflour (cornstarch)

175 ml/6 fl oz/¾ cup chicken stock

Mix together the soy sauce, wine or sherry, sugar, ginger, garlic and spring onions. Add the chicken wings and stir to coat completely. Cover and leave to stand for 1 hour, stirring occasionally. Heat the oil and stir-fry the bamboo shoots for 2 minutes. Remove them from the pan. Drain the chicken and onions, reserving the marinade. Reheat the oil and stir-fry the chicken until browned on all sides. Cover and cook for a further 20 minutes until the chicken is tender. Blend the cornflour with the stock and the reserved marinade. Pour over the chicken and bring to the boil, stirring, until the sauce thickens. Stir in the bamboo shoots and simmer, stirring, for a further 2 minutes.

Royal Chicken Wings

Serves 4

12 chicken wings

250 ml/8 fl oz/1 cup groundnut (peanut) oil

15 ml/1 tbsp granulated sugar

2 spring onions (scallions), cut into chunks

5 slices root ginger

5 ml/1 tsp salt

45 ml/3 tbsp soy sauce

250 ml/8 fl oz/1 cup rice wine or dry sherry

250 ml/8 fl oz/1 cup chicken stock

10 slices bamboo shoots

15 ml/1 tbsp cornflour (cornstarch)

15 ml/1 tbsp water

2.5 ml/½ tsp sesame oil

Blanch the chicken wings in boiling water for 5 minutes then drain well. Heat the oil, add the sugar and stir until melted and golden brown. Add the chicken, spring onions, ginger, salt, soy sauce, wine and stock, bring to the boil and simmer gently for 20 minutes. Add the bamboo shoots and simmer for 2 minutes or until the liquid has almost all evaporated. Blend the cornflour with the water, stir it into the pan and stir until thick. Transfer the chicken wings to a warmed serving plate and serve sprinkled with sesame oil.

Spiced Chicken Wings

Serves 4

30 ml/2 tbsp groundnut (peanut) oil
5 ml/1 tsp salt
2 cloves garlic, crushed
900 g/2 lb chicken wings
30 ml/2 tbsp rice wine or dry sherry
30 ml/2 tbsp soy sauce
30 ml/2 tbsp tomato purée (paste)
15 ml/1 tbsp Worcestershire sauce

Heat the oil, salt and garlic and fry until the garlic turns light golden. Add the chicken wings and fry, stirring frequently, for about 10 minutes until golden brown and almost cooked through. Add the remaining ingredients and stir-fry for about 5 minutes until the chicken is crispy and thoroughly cooked.

Barbecued Chicken Drumsticks

Serves 4

16 chicken drumsticks
30 ml/2 tbsp rice wine or dry sherry
30 ml/2 tbsp wine vinegar
30 ml/2 tbsp olive oil
salt and freshly ground pepper
120 ml/4 fl oz/½ cup orange juice
30 ml/2 tbsp soy sauce
30 ml/2 tbsp honey
15 ml/1 tbsp lemon juice
2 slices ginger root, minced
120 ml/4 fl oz/½ cup chilli sauce

Mix together all the ingredients except the chilli sauce, cover and leave to marinate in the refrigerator overnight. Remove the chicken from the marinade and barbecue or grill (broil) for about 25 minutes, turning and basting with the chilli sauce as you cook.

Hoisin Chicken Drumsticks

Serves 4

8 chicken drumsticks
600 ml/1 pt/2½ cups chicken stock
salt and freshly ground pepper
250 ml/8 fl oz/1 cup hoisin sauce
30 ml/2 tbsp plain (all-purpose) flour
2 eggs, beaten
100 g/4 oz/1 cup breadcrumbs
oil for deep-frying

Place the drumsticks and stock in a pan, bring to the boil, cover and simmer for 20 minutes until cooked. Remove the chicken from the pan and pat dry on kitchen paper. Place the chicken in a bowl and season with salt and pepper. Pour over the hoisin sauce and leave to marinate for 1 hour. Drain. Toss the chicken in the flour then coat in the eggs and breadcrumbs, then in egg and breadcrumbs again. Heat the oil and fry the chicken for about 5 minutes until golden brown. Drain on kitchen paper and serve hot or cold.

Braised Chicken

Serves 4–6

75 ml/5 tbsp groundnut (peanut) oil
1 chicken
3 spring onions (scallions), sliced
3 slices ginger root
120 ml/4 fl oz/½ cup soy sauce
30 ml/2 tbsp rice wine or dry sherry
5 ml/1 tsp sugar

Heat the oil and fry the chicken until browned. Add the spring onions, ginger, soy sauce and wine or sherry, and bring to the boil. Cover and simmer for 30 minutes, turning occasionally. Add the sugar, cover and simmer for a further 30 minutes until the chicken is cooked.

Crispy-Fried Chicken

Serves 4

1 chicken

salt

30 ml/2 tbsp rice wine or dry sherry

3 spring onions (scallions), diced

1 slice ginger root

30 ml/2 tbsp soy sauce

30 ml/2 tbsp sugar

5 ml/1 tsp whole cloves

5 ml/1 tsp salt

5 ml/1 tsp peppercorns

150 ml/¼ pt/generous ½ cup chicken stock

oil for deep-frying

1 lettuce, shredded

4 tomatoes, sliced

½ cucumber, sliced

Rub the chicken with salt and leave to stand for 3 hours. Rinse and place in a bowl. Add the wine or sherry, ginger, soy sauce, sugar, cloves, salt, peppercorns and stock and baste well. Stand the bowl in a steamer, cover and steam for about 2¼ hours until the chicken is thoroughly cooked. Drain. Heat the oil until smoking, then add the chicken and deep-fry until browned. Fry for a further 5 minutes then remove from the oil and drain. Cut into pieces and arrange on a warmed serving plate. Garnish with the lettuce, tomatoes and cucumber and serve with a pepper and salt dip.

Deep-Fried Whole Chicken

Serves 5

1 chicken

10 ml/2 tsp salt

15 ml/1 tbsp rice wine or dry sherry

2 spring onions (scallions), halved

3 slices ginger root, cut into strips

oil for deep-frying

Pat the chicken dry and rub the skin with salt and wine or sherry. Place the spring onions and ginger inside the cavity. Hang the chicken to dry in a cool place for about 3 hours. Heat the oil and place the chicken in a frying basket. Lower gently into the oil and baste continuously inside and out until the chicken is lightly coloured. Remove from the oil and leave to cool slightly while you reheat the oil. Fry again until golden brown. Drain well then chop into pieces.

Five-Spice Chicken

Serves 4–6

1 chicken
120 ml/4 fl oz/½ cup soy sauce
2.5 cm/1 in piece ginger root, minced
1 clove garlic, crushed
15 ml/1 tbsp five-spice powder
30 ml/2 tbsp rice wine or dry sherry
30 ml/2 tbsp honey
2.5 ml/½ tsp sesame oil
oil for deep-frying
30 ml/2 tbsp salt
5 ml/1 tsp freshly ground pepper

Place the chicken in a large saucepan and fill with water to come half way up the thigh. Reserve 15 ml/1 tbsp of the soy sauce and add the remainder to the pan with the ginger, garlic and half the five-spice powder. Bring to the boil, cover and simmer for 5 minutes. Turn off the heat and leave the chicken to stand in the water until the water is lukewarm. Drain.

Cut the chicken in half lengthways and place cut side down in a roasting tin. Mix together the remaining soy sauce and five-spice powder with the wine or sherry, honey and sesame oil. Rub the mixture over the chicken and leave to stand for 2 hours, brushing occasionally with the mixture. Heat the oil and deep-fry the chicken halves for about 15 minutes until golden brown and cooked through. Drain on kitchen paper and cut into serving sized pieces.

Meanwhile, mix the salt and pepper and heat in a dry pan for about 2 minutes. Serve as a dip with the chicken.

Ginger and Spring Onion Chicken

Serves 4

1 chicken

2 slices ginger root, cut into strips

salt and freshly ground pepper

90 ml/4 tbsp groundnut (peanut) oil

8 spring onions (scallions), finely chopped

10 ml/2 tsp white wine vinegar

5 ml/1 tsp soy sauce

Place the chicken in a large saucepan, add half the ginger and pour in enough water almost to cover the chicken. Season with salt and pepper. Bring to the boil, cover and simmer for about 1¼ hours until tender. Leave the chicken to stand in the stock until cool. Drain the chicken and refrigerate until cold. Cut into portions.

Grate the remaining ginger and mix with the oil, spring onions, wine vinegar and soy sauce and salt and pepper. Refrigerate for 1 hour. Place the chicken pieces in a serving bowl and pour over the ginger dressing. Serve with steamed rice.

Poached Chicken

Serves 4

1 chicken
1.2 1/2 pts/5 cups chicken stock or water
30 ml/2 tbsp rice wine or dry sherry
4 spring onions (scallions), chopped
1 slice ginger root
5 ml/1 tsp salt

Place the chicken in a large saucepan with all the remaining ingredients. The stock or water should come half way up the thigh. Bring to the boil, cover and simmer gently for about 1 hour until the chicken is thoroughly cooked. Drain, reserving the stock for soups.

Red-Cooked Chicken

Serves 4

1 chicken

250 ml/8 fl oz/1 cup soy sauce

Place the chicken in a pan, pour over the soy sauce and top up with water almost to cover the chicken. Bring to the boil, cover and simmer for about 1 hour until the chicken is cooked, turning occasionally.

Red-Cooked Spiced Chicken

Serves 4

2 slices ginger root

2 spring onions (scallions)

1 chicken

3 cloves star anise

½ cinnamon stick

15 ml/1 tbsp Szechuan peppercorns

75 ml/5 tbsp soy sauce

75 ml/5 tbsp rice wine or dry sherry

75 ml/5 tbsp sesame oil

15 ml/1 tbsp sugar

Place the ginger and spring onions inside the chicken cavity and place the chicken in a pan. Tie the star anise, cinnamon and peppercorns in a piece of muslin and add it to the pan. Pour over the soy sauce, wine or sherry and sesame oil. Bring to the boil, cover and simmer for about 45 minutes. Add the sugar, cover and simmer for a further 10 minutes until the chicken is cooked through.

Sesame Roast Chicken

Serves 4

50 g/2 oz sesame seeds

1 onion, finely chopped

2 cloves garlic, minced

10 ml/2 tsp salt

1 dried red chilli pepper, crushed

pinch of ground cloves

2.5 ml/½ tsp ground cardamom

2.5 ml/½ tsp ground ginger

75 ml/5 tbsp groundnut (peanut) oil

1 chicken

Mix together all the seasonings and oil and brush over the chicken. Stand it in a roasting tin and add 30 ml/2 tbsp of water to the tin. Roast in a preheated oven at 180°C/350°F/gas mark 4 for about 2 hours, basting and turning the chicken occasionally, until the chicken is golden and cooked through. Add a little more water, if necessary, to prevent burning.

Chicken in Soy Sauce

Serves 4–6

300 ml/½ pt/1¼ cups soy sauce

300 ml/½ pt/1¼ cups rice wine or dry sherry

1 onion, chopped

3 slices root ginger, minced

50 g/2 oz/¼ cup sugar

1 chicken

15 ml/1 tbsp cornflour (cornstarch)

60 ml/4 tbsp water

1 cucumber, peeled and sliced

30 ml/2 tbsp chopped fresh parsley

Mix together the soy sauce, wine or sherry, onion, ginger and sugar in a pan and bring to the boil. Add the chicken, return to the boil, cover and simmer gently for 1 hour, turning the chicken occasionally, until the chicken is cooked. Transfer the chicken to a warmed serving plate and carve. Pour out all but 250 ml/8 fl oz/1 cup of the cooking liquid and bring it back to the boil. Blend the cornflour and water to a paste, stir it into the pan and simmer, stirring, until the sauce clears and thickens. Brush a little of the sauce over the chicken and garnish the chicken with cucumber and parsley. Serve the remaining sauce separately.

Steamed Chicken

Serves 4

1 chicken

45 ml/3 tbsp rice wine or dry sherry

salt

2 slices ginger root

2 spring onions (scallions)

250 ml/8 fl oz/1 cup chicken stock

Place the chicken in an ovenproof bowl and rub with wine or sherry and salt and place the ginger and spring onions inside the cavity. Place the bowl on a rack in a steamer, cover and steam over boiling water for about 1 hour until cooked through. Serve hot or cold.

Steamed Chicken with Anise

Serves 4

250 ml/8 fl oz/1 cup soy sauce

250 ml/8 fl oz/1 cup water

15 ml/1 tbsp brown sugar

4 cloves star anise

1 chicken

Mix the soy sauce, water, sugar and anise in a saucepan and bring to the boil over a gentle heat. Place the chicken in a bowl and baste thoroughly with the mixture inside and out. Reheat the mixture and repeat. Place the chicken in an ovenproof bowl. Place the bowl on a rack in a steamer, cover and steam over boiling water for about 1 hour until cooked through.

Strange-Flavoured Chicken

Serves 4

1 chicken

5 ml/1 tsp minced ginger root

5 ml/1 tsp minced garlic

45 ml/3 tbsp thick soy sauce

5 ml/1 tsp sugar

2.5 ml/½ tsp wine vinegar

10 ml/2 tsp sesame sauce

5 ml/1 tsp freshly ground pepper

10 ml/2 tsp chilli oil

½ lettuce, shredded

15 ml/1 tbsp chopped fresh coriander

Place the chicken in a pan and fill with water to come half way up the chicken legs. Bring to the boil, cover and simmer gently for about 1 hour until the chicken is tender. Remove from the pan and drain well and soak in iced water until the meat cools completely. Drain well and chop into 5 cm/2 in pieces. Mix together all the remaining ingredients and pour over the chicken. Serve garnished with lettuce and coriander.

Crispy Chicken Chunks

Serves 4

100 g/4 oz plain (all-purpose) flour

pinch of salt

15 ml/1 tbsp water

1 egg

350 g/12 oz cooked chicken, cubed

oil for deep-frying

Mix together the flour, salt, water and egg to a fairly stiff batter, adding a little more water if necessary. Dip the chicken pieces into the batter until they are well covered. Heat the oil until very hot and deep-fry the chicken for a few minutes until crispy and golden brown.

Chicken with Green Beans

Serves 4

45 ml/3 tbsp groundnut (peanut) oil
450 g/1 lb cooked chicken, shredded
5 ml/1 tsp salt
2.5 ml/½ tsp freshly ground pepper
225 g/8 oz green beans, cut into pieces
1 stalk celery, diagonally sliced
225 g/8 oz mushrooms, sliced
250 ml/8 fl oz/1 cup chicken stock
30 ml/2 tbsp cornflour (cornstarch)
60 ml/4 tbsp water
10 ml/2 tsp soy sauce

Heat the oil and fry the chicken, salt and pepper until lightly browned. Add the beans, celery and mushrooms and mix well. Add the stock, bring to the boil, cover and simmer for 15 minutes. Mix the cornflour, water and soy sauce to a paste, stir it into the pan and simmer, stirring, until the sauce clears and thickens.

Cooked Chicken with Pineapple

Serves 4

45 ml/3 tbsp groundnut (peanut) oil

225 g/8 oz cooked chicken, diced

salt and freshly ground pepper

2 stalks celery, diagonally sliced

3 slices pineapple, cut into chunks

120 ml/4 fl oz/½ cup chicken stock

15 ml/1 tbsp soy sauce

10 ml/2 tbsp cornflour (cornstarch)

30 ml/2 tbsp water

Heat the oil and fry the chicken until lightly browned. Season with salt and pepper, add the celery and stir-fry for 2 minutes. Add the pineapple, stock and soy sauce and stir for a few minutes until heated through. Mix the cornflour and water to a paste, stir into the pan and simmer, stirring, until the sauce clears and thickens.

Chicken with Peppers and Tomatoes

Serves 4

45 ml/3 tbsp groundnut (peanut) oil
450 g/1 lb cooked chicken, sliced
10 ml/2 tsp salt
5 ml/1 tsp freshly ground pepper
1 green pepper, cut into chunks
4 large tomatoes, skinned and cut into wedges
250 ml/8 fl oz/1 cup chicken stock
30 ml/2 tbsp cornflour (cornstarch)
15 ml/1 tbsp soy sauce
120 ml/4 fl oz/½ cup water

Heat the oil and fry the chicken, salt and pepper until browned. Add the peppers and tomatoes. Pour in the stock, bring to the boil, cover and simmer for 15 minutes. Blend the cornflour, soy sauce and water to a paste, stir it into the pan and simmer, stirring, until the sauce clears and thickens.

Sesame Chicken

Serves 4

450 g/1 lb cooked chicken, cut into strips
2 slices ginger, finely chopped
1 spring onion (scallion), finely chopped
salt and freshly ground pepper
60 ml/4 tbsp rice wine or dry sherry
60 ml/4 tbsp sesame oil
10 ml/2 tsp sugar
5 ml/1 tsp wine vinegar
150 ml/¼ pt/generous ½ cup soy sauce

Arrange the chicken on a serving plate and sprinkle with ginger, spring onion, salt and pepper. Mix together the wine or sherry, sesame oil, sugar, wine vinegar and soy sauce. Pour over the chicken.

Fried Poussins

Serves 4

2 poussins, halved
45 ml/3 tbsp soy sauce
45 ml/3 tbsp rice wine or dry sherry
120 ml/4 fl oz/½ cup groundnut (peanut) oil
1 spring onion (scallion), finely chopped
30 ml/2 tbsp chicken stock
10 ml/2 tsp sugar
5 ml/1 tsp chilli oil
5 ml/1 tsp garlic paste
salt and pepper

Place the poussins in a bowl. Mix the soy sauce and wine or sherry, pour over the poussins, cover and marinate for 2 hours, basting frequently. Heat the oil and fry the poussins for about 20 minutes until cooked through. Remove them from the pan and reheat the oil. Return them to the pan and fry until golden brown. Drain off most of the oil. Mix together the remaining ingredients, add to the pan and heat through quickly. Pour over the poussins before serving.

Turkey with Mangetout

Serves 4

60 ml/4 tbsp groundnut (peanut) oil

2 spring onions (scallions), chopped

2 cloves garlic, crushed

1 slice ginger root, minced

225 g/8 oz turkey breast, cut into strips

225 g/8 oz mangetout (snow peas)

100 g/4 oz bamboo shoots, cut into strips

50 g/2 oz water chestnuts, cut into strips

45 ml/3 tbsp soy sauce

15 ml/1 tbsp rice wine or dry sherry

5 ml/1 tsp sugar

5 ml/1 tsp salt

15 ml/1 tbsp cornflour (cornstarch)

Heat 45 ml/3 tbsp of oil and fry the spring onions, garlic and ginger until lightly browned. Add the turkey and stir-fry for 5 minutes. Remove from the pan and set aside. Heat the remaining oil and stir-fry the mangetout, bamboo shoots and water chestnuts for 3 minutes. Add the soy sauce, wine or sherry, sugar and salt and return the turkey to the pan. Stir-fry for 1 minute.

Mix the cornflour with a little water, stir it into the pan and simmer, stirring, until the sauce clears and thickens.

Turkey with Peppers

Serves 4

4 dried Chinese mushrooms

30 ml/2 tbsp groundnut (peanut) oil

1 Chinese cabbage, cut into strips

350 g/12 oz smoked turkey, cut into strips

1 onion, sliced

1 red pepper, cut into strips

1 green pepper, cut into strips

120 ml/4 fl oz/½ cup chicken stock

30 ml/2 tbsp tomato purée (paste)

45 ml/3 tbsp wine vinegar

30 ml/2 tbsp soy sauce

15 ml/1 tbsp hoisin sauce

10 ml/2 tsp cornflour (cornstarch)

few drops of chilli oil

Soak the mushrooms in warm water for 30 minutes then drain. Discard the stalks and cut the caps into strips. Heat half the oil and stir-fry the cabbage for about 5 minutes or until cooked down. Remove from the pan. Add the turkey and stir-fry for 1 minute. Add the vegetables and stir-fry for 3 minutes. Mix the stock with the tomato purée, wine vinegar and sauces and add to the pan with the cabbage. Mix the cornflour with a little water, stir it into the pan and bring to the boil, stirring. Sprinkle with chilli oil and simmer for 2 minutes, stirring continuously.

Chinese Roast Turkey

Serves 8–10

1 small turkey
600 ml/1 pt/2½ cups hot water
10 ml/2 tsp allspice
500 ml/16 fl oz/2 cups soy sauce
5 ml/1 tsp sesame oil
10 ml/2 tsp salt
45 ml/3 tbsp butter

Place the turkey in a pan and pour over the hot water. Add the remaining ingredients except the butter and leave to stand for 1 hour, turning several times. Remove the turkey from the liquid and brush with butter. Place in a roasting tin, cover loosely with kitchen foil and roast in a preheated oven at 160°C/325°F/gas mark 3 for about 4 hours, basting occasionally with the soy sauce liquid. Remove the foil and allow the skin to crisp for the last 30 minutes of cooking.

Turkey with Walnuts and Mushrooms

Serves 4

450 g/1 lb turkey breast fillet
salt and pepper
juice of 1 orange
15 ml/1 tbsp plain (all-purpose) flour
12 pickled black walnuts with juice
5 ml/1 tsp cornflour (cornstarch)
15 ml/1 tbsp groundnut (peanut) oil
2 spring onions (scallions), diced
225 g/8 oz button mushrooms
45 ml/3 tbsp rice wine or dry sherry
10 ml/2 tsp soy sauce
50 g/2 oz/½ cup butter
25 g/1 oz pine kernels

Cut the turkey into 1 cm/½ in thick slices. Sprinkle with salt, pepper and orange juice and dust with flour. Drain and halve the walnuts, reserving the liquid, and mix the liquid with the cornflour. Heat the oil and stir-fry the turkey until golden brown. Add the spring onions and mushrooms and stir-fry for 2 minutes. Stir in the wine or sherry and soy sauce and simmer for 30 seconds. Add the walnuts to the cornflour mixture then stir them into the pan and bring to the boil. Add the butter in small flakes but do not allow the mixture to boil. Toast the pine kernels in a dry pan until golden. Transfer the turkey mixture to a warmed serving plate and serve garnished with pine kernels.

Duck with Bamboo Shoots

Serves 4

6 dried Chinese mushrooms
1 duck
50 g/2 oz smoked ham, cut into strips
100 g/4 oz bamboo shoots, cut into strips
2 spring onions (scallions), cut into strips
2 slices ginger root, cut into strips
5 ml/1 tsp salt

Soak the mushrooms in warm water for 30 minutes then drain. Discard the stalks and cut the caps into strips. Place all the ingredients in a heatproof bowl and stand in a pan filled with water to come two-thirds of the way up the bowl. Bring to the boil, cover and simmer for about 2 hours until the duck is cooked, topping up with boiling water as necessary.

Duck with Bean Sprouts

Serves 4

225 g/8 oz bean sprouts

45 ml/3 tbsp groundnut (peanut) oil

450 g/1 lb cooked duck meat

15 ml/1 tbsp oyster sauce

15 ml/1 tbsp rice wine or dry sherry

30 ml/2 tbsp water

2.5 ml/½ tsp salt

Blanch the bean sprouts in boiling water for 2 minutes then drain. Heat the oil, stir-fry the bean sprouts for 30 seconds. Add the duck, stir-fry until heated through. Add the remaining ingredients and stir-fry for 2 minutes to blend the flavours. Serve at once.

Braised Duck

Serves 4

4 spring onions (scallions), chopped
1 slice ginger root, minced
120 ml/4 fl oz/½ cup soy sauce
30 ml/2 tbsp rice wine or dry sherry
1 duck
120 ml/4 fl oz/½ cup groundnut (peanut) oil
600 ml/1 pt/2½ cups water
15 ml/1 tbsp brown sugar

Mix together the spring onions, ginger, soy sauce and wine or sherry and rub it over the duck inside and out. Heat the oil and fry the duck until lightly browned on all sides. Drain off the oil. Add the water and the remaining soy sauce mixture, bring to the boil then cover and simmer for 1 hour. Add the sugar then cover and simmer for a further 40 minutes until the duck is tender.

Steamed Duck with Celery

Serves 4

350 g/12 oz cooked duck, sliced
1 head celery
250 ml/8 fl oz/1 cup chicken stock
2.5 ml/½ tsp salt
5 ml/1 tsp sesame oil
1 tomato, cut into wedges

Arrange the duck on a steamer rack. Trim the celery into 7.5 cm/3 in lengths and place in a pan. Pour in the stock, season with salt and place the steamer over the pan. Bring the stock to the boil then simmer gently for about 15 minutes until the celery is tender and the duck heated through. Arrange the duck and celery on a warmed serving plate, sprinkle the celery with sesame oil and serve garnished with tomato wedges.

Duck with Ginger

Serves 4

350 g/12 oz duck breast, thinly sliced

1 egg, lightly beaten

5 ml/1 tsp soy sauce

5 ml/1 tsp cornflour (cornstarch)

5 ml/1 tsp groundnut (peanut) oil

oil for deep-frying

50 g/2 oz bamboo shoots

50 g/2 oz mangetout (snow peas)

2 slices ginger root, chopped

15 ml/1 tbsp water

2.5 ml/½ tsp sugar

2.5 ml/½ tsp rice wine or dry sherry

2.5 ml/½ tsp sesame oil

Mix the duck with the egg, soy sauce, cornflour and oil and leave to stand for 10 minutes. Heat the oil and deep-fry the duck and bamboo shoots until cooked and golden brown. Remove from the pan and drain well. Pour out all but 15 ml/1 tbsp of oil from the pan and stir-fry the duck, bamboo shoots, mangetout, ginger, water, sugar and wine or sherry for 2 minutes. Serve sprinkled with sesame oil.

Duck with Green Beans

Serves 4

1 duck

60 ml/4 tbsp groundnut (peanut) oil

2 cloves garlic, crushed

2.5 ml/½ tsp salt

1 onion, chopped

15 ml/1 tbsp grated root ginger

45 ml/3 tbsp soy sauce

120 ml/4 fl oz/½ cup rice wine or dry sherry

60 ml/4 tbsp tomato ketchup (catsup)

45 ml/3 tbsp wine vinegar

300 ml/½ pt/1¼ cups chicken stock

450 g/1 lb green beans, sliced

pinch of freshly ground pepper

5 drops chilli oil

15 ml/1 tbsp cornflour (cornstarch)

30 ml/2 tbsp water

Chop the duck into 8 or 10 pieces. Heat the oil and fry the duck until golden brown. Transfer to a bowl. Add the garlic, salt, onion, ginger, soy sauce, wine or sherry, tomato ketchup and wine vinegar. Mix, cover and marinate in the refrigerator for 3 hours.

Reheat the oil, add the duck, stock and marinade, bring to the boil, cover and simmer for 1 hour. Add the beans, cover and simmer for 15 minutes. Add the pepper and chilli oil. Mix the cornflour with the water, stir it into the pan and simmer, stirring, until the sauce thickens.

Deep-Fried Steamed Duck

Serves 4

1 duck
salt and freshly ground pepper
oil for deep-frying
hoisin sauce

Season the duck with salt and pepper and place in a heatproof bowl. Stand in a pan filled with water to come two-thirds of the way up the bowl, bring to the boil, cover and simmer for about 1½ hours until the duck is tender. Drain and leave to cool.

Heat the oil and deep-fry the duck until crispy and golden brown. Remove and drain well. Chop into bite-sized pieces and serve with hoisin sauce.

Duck with Exotic Fruits

Serves 4

4 duck breast fillets, cut into strips

2.5 ml/½ tsp five-spice powder

30 ml/2 tbsp soy sauce

15 ml/1 tbsp sesame oil

15 ml/1 tbsp groundnut (peanut) oil

3 stalks celery, diced

2 slices pineapple, diced

100 g/4 oz melon, diced

100 g/4 oz lychees, halved

130 ml/4 fl oz/½ cup chicken stock

30 ml/2 tbsp tomato purée (paste)

30 ml/2 tbsp hoisin sauce

10 ml/2 tsp wine vinegar

pinch of brown sugar

Place the duck in a bowl. Mix the five-spice powder, soy sauce and sesame oil, pour over the duck and marinate for 2 hours, stirring occasionally. Heat the oil and stir-fry the duck for 8 minutes. Remove from the pan. Add the celery and fruits and stir-fry for 5 minutes. Return the duck to the pan with the remaining ingredients, bring to the boil and simmer, stirring, for 2 minutes before serving.

Braised Duck with Chinese Leaves

Serves 4

1 duck

30 ml/2 tbsp rice wine or dry sherry

30 ml/2 tbsp hoisin sauce

15 ml/1 tbsp cornflour (cornstarch)

5 ml/1 tsp salt

5 ml/1 tsp sugar

60 ml/4 tbsp groundnut (peanut) oil

4 spring onions (scallions), chopped

2 cloves garlic, crushed

1 slice ginger root, minced

75 ml/5 tbsp soy sauce

600 ml/1 pt/2½ cups water

225 g/8 oz Chinese leaves, shredded

Cut the duck into about 6 pieces. Mix together the wine or sherry, hoisin sauce, cornflour, salt and sugar and rub over the duck. Leave to stand for 1 hour. Heat the oil and fry the spring onions, garlic and ginger for a few seconds. Add the duck and fry until lightly browned on all sides. Drain off any excess fat. Pour in the soy sauce and water, bring to the boil, cover and simmer for about 30 minutes. Add the Chinese leaves, cover again and simmer for a further 30 minutes until the duck is tender.

Drunken Duck

Serves 4

2 spring onions (scallions), chopped
2 cloves garlic, chopped
1.5 l/2½ pts/6 cups water
1 duck
450 ml/¾ pt/2 cups rice wine or dry sherry

Place the spring onions, garlic and water in a large pan and bring to the boil. Add the duck, return to the boil, cover and simmer for 45 minutes. Drain well, reserving the liquid for stock. Leave the duck to cool then refrigerate overnight. Cut the duck into pieces and place them in a large screw-top jar. Pour over the wine or sherry and chill for about 1 week before draining and serving cold.

Five-Spice Duck

Serves 4

150 ml/¼ pt/generous ½ cup rice wine or dry sherry

150 ml/¼ pt/generous ½ cup soy sauce

1 duck

10 ml/2 tsp five-spice powder

Bring the wine or sherry and soy sauce to the boil. Add the duck and simmer, turning for about 5 minutes. Remove the duck from the pan and rub the five-spice powder into the skin. Return the bird to the pan and add enough water to half cover the duck. Bring to the boil, cover and simmer for about 1½ hours until the duck is tender, turning and basting frequently. Chop the duck into 5 cm/2 in pieces and serve hot or cold.

Stir-Fried Duck with Ginger

Serves 4

1 duck

2 slices ginger root, shredded

2 spring onions (scallions), chopped

15 ml/1 tbsp cornflour (cornstarch)

30 ml/2 tbsp soy sauce

30 ml/2 tbsp rice wine or dry sherry

2.5 ml/½ tsp salt

45 ml/3 tbsp groundnut (peanut) oil

Remove the meat from the bones and cut into pieces. Mix the meat with all the remaining ingredients except the oil. Leave to stand for 1 hour. Heat the oil and stir-fry the duck with the marinade for about 15 minutes until the duck is tender.

Duck with Ham and Leeks

Serves 4

1 duck

450 g/1 lb smoked ham

2 leeks

2 slices ginger root, minced

45 ml/3 tbsp rice wine or dry sherry

45 ml/3 tbsp soy sauce

2.5 ml/½ tsp salt

Place the duck in a pan and just cover with cold water. Bring to the boil, cover and simmer for about 20 minutes. Drain and reserve 450 ml/¾ pts/2 cups of stock. Let the duck cool slightly then cut the meat from the bones and cut it into 5 cm/2 in squares. Cut the ham into similar pieces. Cut off long pieces of leek and roll a slice of duck and ham inside the leaf and tie with string. Place in a heatproof bowl. Add the ginger, wine or sherry, soy sauce and salt to the reserved stock and pour it over the duck rolls. Place the bowl in a pan filled with water to come two-thirds of the way up the sides of the bowl. Bring to the boil, cover and simmer for about 1 hour until the duck is tender.

Honey-Roast Duck

Serves 4

1 duck

salt

3 cloves garlic, crushed

3 spring onions (scallions), minced

45 ml/3 tbsp soy sauce

45 ml/3 tbsp rice wine or dry sherry

45 ml/3 tbsp honey

200 ml/7 fl oz/scant 1 cup boiling water

Pat the duck dry and rub with salt inside and out. Mix the garlic, spring onions, soy sauce and wine or sherry then divide the mixture in half. Mix the honey into one half and rub over the duck then leave it to dry. Add the water to the remaining honey mixture. Pour the soy sauce mixture into the cavity of the duck and stand it on a rack in a roasting tin with a little water in the bottom. Roast in a preheated oven at 180°C/350°F/gas mark 4 for about 2 hours until the duck is tender, basting throughout cooking with the remaining honey mixture.

Moist Roast Duck

Serves 4

6 spring onions (scallions), chopped
2 slices ginger root, minced
1 duck
2.5 ml/½ tsp ground anise
15 ml/1 tbsp sugar
45 ml/3 tbsp rice wine or dry sherry
60 ml/4 tbsp soy sauce
250 ml/8 fl oz/1 cup water

Place half the spring onions and ginger in a large heavy-based pan. Place the remainder in the cavity of the duck and add it to the pan. Add all the remaining ingredients except the hoisin sauce, bring to the boil, cover and simmer for about 1½ hours, turning occasionally. Remove the duck from the pan and leave it to dry for about 4 hours.

Place the duck on a rack in a roasting tin filled with a little cold water. Roast in a preheated oven at 230°C/450°F/gas mark 8 for 15 minutes then turn it over and roast for a further 10 minutes until crispy. Meanwhile, reheat the reserved liquid and pour over the duck to serve.

Stir-Fried Duck with Mushrooms

Serves 4

1 duck

75 ml/5 tbsp groundnut (peanut) oil

45 ml/3 tbsp rice wine or dry sherry

15 ml/1 tbsp soy sauce

15 ml/1 tbsp sugar

5 ml/1 tsp salt

pinch of pepper

2 cloves garlic, crushed

225 g/8 oz mushrooms, halved

600 ml/1 pt/2½ cups chicken stock

15 ml/1 tbsp cornflour (cornstarch)

30 ml/2 tbsp water

5 ml/1 tsp sesame oil

Chop the duck into 5 cm/2 in pieces. Heat 45 ml/3 tbsp of oil and fry the duck until lightly browned on all sides. Add the wine or sherry, soy sauce, sugar, salt and pepper and stir-fry for 4 minutes. Remove from the pan. Heat the remaining oil and fry the garlic until lightly browned. Add the mushrooms and stir until coated in oil then return the duck mixture to the pan and add the stock. Bring to the boil, cover and simmer for about 1 hour until the duck is tender. Mix the cornflour and water to a paste then stir it into the mixture and simmer, stirring, until the sauce thickens. Sprinkle with sesame oil and serve.

Duck with Two Mushrooms

Serves 4

6 dried Chinese mushrooms
1 duck
750 ml/1¼ pts/3 cups chicken stock
45 ml/3 tbsp rice wine or dry sherry
5 ml/1 tsp salt
100 g/4 oz bamboo shoots, cut into strips
100 g/4 oz button mushrooms

Soak the mushrooms in warm water for 30 minutes then drain. Discard the stalks and halve the caps. Place the duck in a large heatproof bowl with the stock, wine or sherry and salt and stand in a pan filled with water to come two-thirds up the sides of the bowl. Bring to the boil, cover and simmer for about 2 hours until the duck is tender. Remove from the pan and cut the meat from the bone. Transfer the cooking liquid to a separate pan. Arrange the bamboo shoots and both types of mushrooms in the bottom of the steamer bowl, replace the duck meat, cover and steam for a further 30 minutes. Bring the cooking liquid to the boil and pour over the duck to serve.

Braised Duck with Onions

Serves 4

4 dried Chinese mushrooms

1 duck

90 ml/6 tbsp soy sauce

60 ml/4 tbsp groundnut (peanut) oil

1 spring onion (scallion), chopped

1 slice ginger root, minced

45 ml/3 tbsp rice wine or dry sherry

450 g/1 lb onions, sliced

100 g/4 oz bamboo shoots, sliced

15 ml/1 tbsp brown sugar

15 ml/1 tbsp cornflour (cornstarch)

45 ml/3 tbsp water

Soak the mushrooms in warm water for 30 minutes then drain. Discard the stalks and slice the caps. Rub 15 ml/1 tbsp of soy sauce into the duck. Reserve 15 ml/1 tbsp of oil, heat the remaining oil and fry the spring onion and ginger until lightly browned. Add the duck and fry until lightly browned on all sides. Pour off any excess fat. Add the wine or sherry, remaining soy sauce to the pan and just enough water almost to cover the duck.

Bring to the boil, cover and simmer for 1 hour, turning occasionally.

Heat the reserved oil and fry the onions until softened. Remove from the heat and stir in the bamboo shoots and mushrooms then add them to the duck, cover and simmer for a further 30 minutes until the duck is tender. Remove the duck from the pan, cut into serving pieces and arrange on a warmed serving plate. Bring the liquids in the pan to the boil, add the sugar and cornflour and simmer, stirring, until the mixture boils and thickens. Pour over the duck to serve.

Duck with Orange

Serves 4

1 duck

3 spring onions (scallions), cut into chunks

2 slices ginger root, cut into strips

1 slice orange rind

salt and freshly ground pepper

Place the duck in a large pan, just cover with water and bring to the boil. Add the spring onions, ginger and orange rind, cover and simmer for about 1½ hours until the duck is tender. Season with salt and pepper, drain and serve.

Orange-Roast Duck

Serves 4

1 duck

2 cloves garlic, halved

45 ml/3 tbsp groundnut (peanut) oil

1 onion

1 orange

120 ml/4 fl oz/½ cup rice wine or dry sherry

2 slices ginger root, minced

5 ml/1 tsp salt

Rub the garlic over the duck inside and out then brush it with oil. Pierce the peeled onion with a fork, place it and the unpeeled orange inside the duck cavity and seal with a skewer. Stand the duck on a rack over a roasting tin filled with a little hot water and roast in a preheated oven at 160°C/325°F/gas mark 3 for about 2 hours. Discard the liquids and return the duck to the roasting tin. Pour over the wine or sherry and sprinkle with the ginger and salt. Return to the oven for a further 30 minutes. Discard the onion and orange and cut the duck into serving pieces. Pour the pan juices over the duck to serve.

Duck with Pears and Chestnuts

Serves 4

225 g/8 oz chestnuts, shelled

1 duck

45 ml/3 tbsp groundnut (peanut) oil

250 ml/8 fl oz/1 cup chicken stock

45 ml/3 tbsp soy sauce

15 ml/1 tbsp rice wine or dry sherry

5 ml/1 tsp salt

1 slice ginger root, minced

1 large pear, peeled and thickly sliced

15 ml/1 tbsp sugar

Boil the chestnuts for 15 minutes then drain. Chop the duck into 5 cm/2 in pieces. Heat the oil and fry the duck until lightly browned on all sides. Drain off any excess oil then add the stock, soy sauce, wine or sherry, salt and ginger. Bring to the boil, cover and simmer for 25 minutes, stirring occasionally. Add the chestnuts, cover and simmer for a further 15 minutes. Sprinkle the pear with sugar, add to the pan and simmer for about 5 minutes until heated through.

Peking Duck

Serves 6

1 duck

250 ml/8 fl oz/1 cup water

120 ml/4 fl oz/½ cup honey

120 ml/4 fl oz/½ cup sesame oil

For the pancakes:

250 ml/8 fl oz/1 cup water

225 g/8 oz/2 cups plain (all-purpose) flour

groundnut (peanut) oil for frying

For the dips:

120 ml/4 fl oz/½ cup hoisin sauce

30 ml/2 tbsp brown sugar

30 ml/2 tbsp soy sauce

5 ml/1 tsp sesame oil

6 spring onions (scallions), sliced lengthways

1 cucumber, cut into strips

The duck should be whole with the skin intact. Tie the neck tightly with string and sew up or skewer the bottom opening. Cut a small slit in the side of the neck, insert a straw and blow air under the skin until it is inflated. Suspend the duck over a basin and leave to hang for 1 hour.

Bring a pan of water to the boil, insert the duck and boil for 1 minute then remove and dry well. Bring the water to the boil and stir in the honey. Rub the mixture over the duck skin until it is saturated. Hang the duck over a basin in a cool, airy place for about 8 hours until the skin is hard.

Suspend the duck or place on a rack over a roasting tin and roast in a preheated oven at 180°C/350°F/gas mark 4 for about 1½ hours, basting regularly with sesame oil.

To make the pancakes, boil the water then gradually add the flour. Knead lightly until the dough is soft, cover with a damp cloth and leave to stand for 15 minutes. Roll out on a floured surface and shape into a long cylinder. Cut into 2.5 cm/1 in slices then flatten until about 5 mm/¼ in thick and brush the tops with oil. Stack in pairs with the oiled surfaces touching and dust the outsides lightly with flour. Roll out the pairs to about 10 cm/4 in across and cook in pairs for about 1 minute on each side until lightly browned. Separate and stack until ready to serve.

Prepare the dips by mixing half the hoisin sauce with the sugar and mixing the remaining hoisin sauce with the soy sauce and sesame oil.

Remove the duck from the oven, cut off the skin and cut it into squares, and cube the meat. Arrange on separate plates and serve with the pancakes, dips and accompaniments.

Braised Duck with Pineapple

Serves 4

1 duck
400 g/14 oz canned pineapple chunks in syrup
45 ml/3 tbsp soy sauce
5 ml/1 tsp salt
pinch of freshly ground pepper

Place the duck in a heavy-based pan, just cover with water, bring to the boil then cover and simmer for 1 hour. Drain the pineapple syrup into the pan with the soy sauce, salt and pepper, cover and simmer for a further 30 minutes. Add the pineapple pieces and simmer for a further 15 minutes until the duck is tender.

Stir-Fried Duck with Pineapple

Serves 4

1 duck
45 ml/3 tbsp cornflour (cornstarch)
45 ml/3 tbsp soy sauce
225 g/8 oz canned pineapple in syrup
45 ml/3 tbsp groundnut (peanut) oil
2 slices ginger root, cut into strips
15 ml/1 tbsp rice wine or dry sherry
5 ml/1 tsp salt

Cut the meat from the bone and cut it into pieces. Mix the soy sauce with 30 ml/2 tbsp of cornflour and mix into the duck until well coated. Leave to stand for 1 hour, stirring occasionally. Crush the pineapple and syrup and heat gently in a pan. Mix the remaining cornflour with a little water, stir into the pan and simmer, stirring, until the sauce thickens. Keep warm. Heat the oil and fry the ginger until lightly browned then discard the ginger. Add the duck and stir-fry until lightly browned on all sides. Add the wine or sherry and salt and stir-fry for a further few minutes until the duck is cooked. Arrange the duck on a warmed serving plate, pour over the sauce and serve at once.

Pineapple and Ginger Duck

Serves 4

1 duck
100 g/4 oz preserved ginger in syrup
200 g/7 oz canned pineapple chunks in syrup
5 ml/1 tsp salt
15 ml/1 tbsp cornflour (cornstarch)
30 ml/2 tbsp water

Place the duck in a heatproof bowl and stand it in a pan filled with water to come two-thirds of the way up the sides of the bowl. Bring to the boil, cover and simmer for about 2 hours until the duck is tender. Remove the duck and leave to cool slightly. Remove the skin and bone and cut the duck into pieces. Arrange on a serving plate and keep them warm.

Drain the syrup from the ginger and pineapple into a pan, add the salt, cornflour and water. Bring to the boil, stirring and simmer for a few minutes, stirring, until the sauce clears and thickens. Add the ginger and pineapple, stir through then pour over the duck to serve.

Duck with Pineapple and Lychees

Serves 4

4 duck breasts

15 ml/1 tbsp soy sauce

1 clove star anise

1 slice ginger root

groundnut (peanut) oil for deep-frying

90 ml/6 tbsp wine vinegar

100 g/4 oz/½ cup brown sugar

250 ml/8 fl oz/½ cup chicken stock

15 ml/1 tbsp tomato ketchup (catsup)

200 g/7 oz canned pineapple chunks in syrup

15 ml/1 tbsp cornflour (cornstarch)

6 canned lychees

6 maraschino cherries

Place the ducks, soy sauce, anise and ginger in a saucepan and just cover with cold water. Bring to the boil, skim, then cover and simmer for about 45 minutes until the duck is cooked. Drain and pat dry. Deep-fry in hot oil until crispy.

Meanwhile, mix the wine vinegar, sugar, stock, tomato ketchup and 30 ml/2 tbsp of the pineapple syrup in a pan, bring to the boil and simmer for about 5 minutes until thick. Stir in the fruit and heat through before pouring over the duck to serve.

Duck with Pork and Chestnuts

Serves 4

6 dried Chinese mushrooms
1 duck
225 g/8 oz chestnuts, shelled
225 g/8 oz lean pork, cubed
3 spring onions (scallions), chopped
1 slice ginger root, minced
250 ml/8 fl oz/1 cup soy sauce
900 ml/1½ pts/3¾ cups water

Soak the mushrooms in warm water for 30 minutes then drain. Discard the stalks and slice the caps. Place in a large pan with all the remaining ingredients, bring to the boil, cover and simmer for about 1½ hours until the duck is cooked.

Duck with Potatoes

Serves 4

75 ml/5 tbsp groundnut (peanut) oil

1 duck

3 cloves garlic, crushed

30 ml/2 tbsp black bean sauce

10 ml/2 tsp salt

1.2 l/2 pts/5 cups water

2 leeks, thickly sliced

15 ml/1 tbsp sugar

45 ml/3 tbsp soy sauce

60 ml/4 tbsp rice wine or dry sherry

1 clove star anise

900 g/2 lb potatoes, thickly sliced

½ head Chinese leaves

15 ml/1 tbsp cornflour (cornstarch)

30 ml/2 tbsp water

sprigs flat-leaf parsley

Heat 60 ml/4 tbsp of oil and fry the duck until browned on all sides. Tie or sew up the neck end and stand the duck, neck down, in a deep bowl. Heat the remaining oil and fry the garlic until lightly browned. Add the black bean sauce and salt and fry for 1 minute. Add the water, leeks, sugar, soy sauce, wine or sherry and star anise and bring to the boil. Pour 120 ml/8 fl oz/1 cup of the mixture into the duck cavity and tie or sew up to secure. Bring the remaining mixture in the pan to the boil. Add the duck and potatoes, cover and simmer for 40 minutes, turning the duck once. Arrange the Chinese leaves on a serving plate. Remove the duck from the pan, chop into 5 cm/2 in pieces and arrange on the serving plate with the potatoes. Mix the cornflour to a paste with the water, stir it into the pan and simmer, stirring, until the sauce thickens. Pour over the duck and serve garnished with parsley.

Red-Cooked Duck

Serves 4

1 duck

4 spring onions (scallions), cut into chunks

2 slices ginger root, cut into strips

90 ml/6 tbsp soy sauce

45 ml/3 tbsp rice wine or dry sherry

10 ml/2 tsp salt

10 ml/2 tsp sugar

Place the duck in a heavy pan, just cover with water and bring to the boil. Add the spring onions, ginger, wine or sherry and salt, cover and simmer for about 1 hour. Add the sugar and simmer for a further 45 minutes until the duck is tender. Slice the duck on to a serving plate and serve hot or cold, with or without the sauce.

Rice Wine Roast Duck

Serves 4

1 duck

500 ml/14 fl oz/1¾ cups rice wine or dry sherry

5 ml/1 tsp salt

45 ml/3 tbsp soy sauce

Place the duck in a heavy-based pan with the sherry and salt, bring to the boil, cover and simmer for 20 minutes. Drain the duck, reserving the liquid, and rub it with soy sauce. Place on a rack in a roasting tin filled with a little hot water and roast in a preheated oven at 180°C/350°F/gas mark 4 for about 1 hour, basting regularly with the reserved wine liquid.

Steamed Duck with Rice Wine

Serves 4

1 duck

4 spring onions (scallions), halved

1 slice ginger root, chopped

250 ml/8 fl oz/1 cup rice wine or dry sherry

30 ml/2 tbsp soy sauce

pinch of salt

Blanch the duck in boiling water for 5 minutes then drain. Place in a heatproof bowl with the remaining ingredients. Stand the bowl in a pan filled with water to come two-thirds of the way up the sides of the bowl. Bring to the boil, cover and simmer for about 2 hours until the duck is tender. Discard the spring onions and ginger before serving.

Savoury Duck

Serves 4

45 ml/3 tbsp groundnut (peanut) oil
4 duck breasts
3 spring onions (scallions), sliced
2 cloves garlic, crushed
1 slice ginger root, chopped
250 ml/8 fl oz/1 cup soy sauce
30 ml/2 tbsp rice wine or dry sherry
30 ml/2 tbsp brown sugar
5 ml/1 tsp salt
450 ml/¾ pt/2 cups water
15 ml/1 tbsp cornflour (cornstarch)

Heat the oil and fry the duck breasts until golden brown. Add the spring onions, garlic and ginger and fry for 2 minutes. Add the soy sauce, wine or sherry, sugar and salt and mix well. Add the water, bring to the boil, cover and simmer for about 1½ hours until the meat is very tender. Mix the cornflour with a little water then stir it into the pan and simmer, stirring, until the sauce thickens.

Savoury Duck with Green Beans

Serves 4

45 ml/3 tbsp groundnut (peanut) oil
4 duck breasts
3 spring onions (scallions), sliced
2 cloves garlic, crushed
1 slice ginger root, chopped
250 ml/8 fl oz/1 cup soy sauce
30 ml/2 tbsp rice wine or dry sherry
30 ml/2 tbsp brown sugar
5 ml/1 tsp salt
450 ml/¾ pt/2 cups water
225 g/8 oz green beans
15 ml/1 tbsp cornflour (cornstarch)

Heat the oil and fry the duck breasts until golden brown. Add the spring onions, garlic and ginger and fry for 2 minutes. Add the soy sauce, wine or sherry, sugar and salt and mix well. Add the water, bring to the boil, cover and simmer for about 45 minutes. Add the beans, cover and simmer for a further 20 minutes. Mix the cornflour with a little water then stir it into the pan and simmer, stirring, until the sauce thickens.

Slow-Cooked Duck

Serves 4

1 duck

50 g/2 oz/½ cup cornflour (cornstarch)

oil for deep-frying

2 cloves garlic, crushed

30 ml/2 tbsp rice wine or dry sherry

30 ml/2 tbsp soy sauce

5 ml/1 tsp grated ginger root

750 ml/1¼ pts/3 cups chicken stock

4 dried Chinese mushrooms

225 g/8 oz bamboo shoots, sliced

225 g/8 oz water chestnuts, sliced

10 ml/2 tsp sugar

pinch of pepper

5 spring onions (scallions), sliced

Cut the duck into serving-size pieces. Reserve 30 ml/2 tbsp of cornflour and coat the duck in the remaining cornflour. Dust off the excess. Heat the oil and fry the garlic and duck until lightly browned. Remove from the pan and drain on kitchen paper. Place the duck in a large pan. Mix together the wine or sherry, 15 ml/1 tbsp of soy sauce and the ginger. Add to the pan and cook over a high heat for 2 minutes. Add half the stock, bring to the boil, cover and simmer for about 1 hour until the duck is tender.

Meanwhile, soak the mushrooms in warm water for 30 minutes then drain. Discard the stalks and slice the caps. Add the mushrooms, bamboo shoots and water chestnuts to the duck and cook, stirring frequently, for 5 minutes. Skim off any fat from the liquid. Blend the remaining stock, cornflour and soy sauce with the sugar and pepper and stir into the pan. Bring to the boil, stirring, then simmer for about 5 minutes until the sauce thickens. Transfer to a warmed serving bowl and serve garnished with spring onions.

Stir-Fried Duck

Serves 4

1 egg white, lightly beaten

20 ml/1½ tbsp cornflour (cornstarch)

salt

450 g/1 lb duck breasts, thinly sliced

45 ml/3 tbsp groundnut (peanut) oil

2 spring onions (scallions), cut into strips

1 green pepper, cut into strips

5 ml/1 tsp rice wine or dry sherry

75 ml/5 tbsp chicken stock

2.5 ml/½ tsp sugar

Beat the egg white with 15 ml/1 tbsp of cornflour and a pinch of salt. Add the sliced duck and mix until the duck is coated. Heat the oil and fry the duck until cooked through and golden. Remove the duck from the pan and drain off all but 30 ml/2 tbsp of the oil. Add the spring onions and pepper and stir-fry for 3 minutes. Add the wine or sherry, stock and sugar and bring to the boil. Mix the remaining cornflour with a little water, stir it into the sauce and simmer, stirring, until the sauce thickens. Stir in the duck, heat through and serve.

Duck with Sweet Potatoes

Serves 4

1 duck

250 ml/8 fl oz/1 cup groundnut (peanut) oil

225 g/8 oz sweet potatoes, peeled and cubed

2 cloves garlic, crushed

1 slice ginger root, minced

2.5 ml/½ tsp cinnamon

2.5 ml/½ tsp ground cloves

pinch of ground anise

5 ml/1 tsp sugar

15 ml/1 tbsp soy sauce

250 ml/8 fl oz/1 cup chicken stock

15 ml/1 tbsp cornflour (cornstarch)

30 ml/2 tbsp water

Chop the duck into 5 cm/2 in pieces. Heat the oil and deep-fry the potatoes until golden brown. Remove them from the pan and drain off all but 30 ml/2 tbsp of oil. Add the garlic and ginger and stir-fry for 30 seconds. Add the duck and fry until lightly browned on all sides. Add the spices, sugar, soy sauce and stock and bring to the boil. Add the potatoes, cover and simmer for about 20 minutes until the duck is tender. Blend the cornflour to a paste with the water then stir it into the pan and simmer, stirring, until the sauce thickens.

Sweet and Sour Duck

Serves 4

1 duck

1.2 l/2 pts/5 cups chicken stock

2 onions

2 carrots

2 cloves garlic, sliced

15 ml/1 tbsp pickling spice

10 ml/2 tsp salt

10 ml/2 tsp groundnut (peanut) oil

6 spring onions (scallions), chopped

1 mango, peeled and cubed

12 lychees, halved

15 ml/1 tbsp cornflour (cornstarch)

15 ml/1 tbsp wine vinegar

10 ml/2 tsp tomato purée (paste)

15 ml/1 tbsp soy sauce

5 ml/1 tsp five-spice powder

300 ml/½ pt/1¼ cups chicken stock

Arrange the duck in a steam basket over a pan containing the stock, onions, carrots, garlic, pickling spice and salt. Cover and steam for 2½ hours. Cool the duck, cover and chill for 6 hours.

Remove the meat from the bones and cut it into cubes. Heat the oil and fry the duck and spring onions until crisp. Stir in the remaining ingredients, bring to the boil and simmer for 2 minutes, stirring, until the sauce thickens.

Tangerine Duck

Serves 4

1 duck
60 ml/4 tbsp groundnut (peanut) oil
1 piece dried tangerine peel
900 ml/1½ pts/3¾ cups chicken stock
5 ml/1 tsp salt

Hang the duck to dry for 2 hours. Heat half the oil and fry the duck until lightly browned. Transfer to a large heatproof bowl. Heat the remaining oil and fry the tangerine peel for 2 minutes then place it inside the duck. Pour the stock over the duck and season with salt. Place the bowl on a rack in a steamer, cover and steam for about 2 hours until the duck is tender.

Duck with Vegetables

Serves 4

1 large duck, chopped into 16 pieces

salt

300 ml/½ pt/1¼ cups water

300 ml/½ pt/1¼ cups dry white wine

120 ml/4 fl oz/½ cup wine vinegar

45 ml/3 tbsp soy sauce

30 ml/2 tbsp plum sauce

30 ml/2 tbsp hoisin sauce

5 ml/1 tsp five-spice powder

6 spring onions (scallions), chopped

2 carrots, chopped

5 cm/2 in white radish, chopped

50 g/2 oz Chinese cabbage, diced

freshly ground pepper

5 ml/1 tsp sugar

Put the duck pieces in a bowl, sprinkle with salt and add the water and wine. Add the wine vinegar, soy sauce, plum sauce, hoisin sauce and five-spice powder, bring to the boil, cover and simmer for about 1 hour. Add the vegetables to the pan, remove the lid and simmer for a further 10 minutes. Season with salt, pepper and sugar then leave to cool. Cover and refrigerate overnight. Skim off any fat then reheat the duck in the sauce for 20 minutes.

Stir-Fried Duck with Vegetables

Serves 4

4 dried Chinese mushrooms
1 duck
10 ml/2 tsp cornflour (cornstarch)
15 ml/1 tbsp soy sauce
45 ml/3 tbsp groundnut (peanut) oil
100 g/4 oz bamboo shoots, cut into strips
50 g/2 oz water chestnuts, cut into strips
120 ml/4 fl oz/½ cup chicken stock
15 ml/1 tbsp rice wine or dry sherry
5 ml/1 tsp salt

Soak the mushrooms in warm water for 30 minutes then drain. Discard the stalks and dice the caps. Remove the meat from the bones and cut into pieces. Mix the cornflour and soy sauce, add to the duck meat and leave to stand for 1 hour. Heat the oil and fry the duck until lightly browned on all sides. Remove from the pan. Add the mushrooms, bamboo shoots and water chestnuts to the pan and stir-fry for 3 minutes. Add the stock, wine or sherry and salt, bring to the boil and simmer for 3 minutes. Return the duck to the pan, cover and simmer for a further 10 minutes until the duck is tender.

White-Cooked Duck

Serves 4

1 slice ginger root, chopped
250 ml/8 fl oz/1 cup rice wine or dry sherry
salt and freshly ground pepper
1 duck
3 spring onions (scallions), chopped
5 ml/1 tsp salt
100 g/4 oz bamboo shoots, sliced
100 g/4 oz smoked ham, sliced

Mix the ginger, 15 ml/1 tbsp wine or sherry, a little salt and pepper. Rub over the duck and leave to stand for 1 hour. Place the bird in a heavy-based pan with the marinade and add the spring onions and salt. Add enough cold water just to cover the duck, bring to the boil, cover and simmer for about 2 hours until the duck is tender. Add the bamboo shoots and ham and simmer for a further 10 minutes.

Duck with Wine

Serves 4

1 duck

15 ml/1 tbsp yellow bean sauce

1 onion, sliced

1 bottle dry white wine

Rub the duck inside and out with the yellow bean sauce. Place the onion inside the cavity. Bring the wine to the boil in a large pan, add the duck, return to the boil, cover and simmer as gently as possible for about 3 hours until the duck is tender. Drain and slice to serve.

Wine-Vapour Duck

Serves 4

1 duck

celery salt

200 ml/7 fl oz/scant 1 cup rice wine or dry sherry

30 ml/2 tbsp chopped fresh parsley

Rub the duck with celery salt inside and out then place it in a deep ovenproof dish. Place an ovenproof cup containing the wine into the cavity of the duck. Place the dish on a rack in a steamer, cover and steam over boiling water for about 2 hours until the duck is tender.

Fried Pheasant

Serves 4

900 g/2 lb pheasant

30 ml/2 tbsp soy sauce

4 eggs, beaten

120 ml/4 fl oz/½ cup groundnut (peanut) oil

Bone the pheasant and slice the meat. Mix with the soy sauce and leave to stand for 30 minutes. Drain the pheasant then dip it in the eggs. Heat the oil and fry the pheasant quickly until golden brown. Drain well before serving.

Pheasant with Almonds

Serves 4

45 ml/3 tbsp groundnut (peanut) oil
2 spring onions (scallions), chopped
1 slice ginger root, minced
225 g/8 oz pheasant, very thinly sliced
50 g/2 oz ham, shredded
30 ml/2 tbsp soy sauce
30 ml/2 tbsp rice wine or dry sherry
5 ml/1 tsp sugar
5 ml/1 tsp freshly ground pepper
2.5 ml/½ tsp salt
100 g/4 oz/1 cup flaked almonds

Heat the oil and fry the spring onions and ginger until lightly browned. Add the pheasant and ham and stir-fry for 5 minutes until almost cooked. Add the soy sauce, wine or sherry, sugar, pepper and salt and stir-fry for 2 minutes. Add the almonds and stir-fry for 1 minute until the ingredients are thoroughly blended.

Venison with Dried Mushrooms

Serves 4

8 dried Chinese mushrooms
450 g/1 lb venison fillet, cut into strips
15 ml/1 tbsp juniper berries, ground
15 ml/1 tbsp sesame oil
30 ml/2 tbsp soy sauce
30 ml/2 tbsp hoisin sauce
5 ml/1 tsp five-spice powder
30 ml/2 tbsp groundnut (peanut) oil
6 spring onions (scallions), chopped
30 ml/2 tbsp honey
30 ml/2 tbsp wine vinegar

Soak the mushrooms in warm water for 30 minutes then drain. Discard the stalks and slice the caps. Place the venison in a bowl. Mix the juniper berries, sesame oil, soy sauce, hoisin sauce and five-spice powder, pour over the venison and marinate for at least 3 hours, stirring occasionally. Heat the oil and stir-fry the meat for 8 minutes until cooked. Remove from the pan. Add the spring onions and mushrooms to the pan and stir-fry for 3 minutes. Return the meat to the pan with the honey and wine vinegar and heat through, stirring.

Salted Eggs

Makes 6

1.2 l/2 pts/5 cups water

100 g/4 oz rock salt

6 duck eggs

Bring the water to the boil with the salt and stir until the salt has dissolved. Leave to cool. Pour the salt water into a large jar, add the eggs, cover and leave to stand for 1 month. Hard-boil the eggs before steaming with rice.

Soy Eggs

Serves 4

4 eggs

120 ml/4 fl oz/½ cup soy sauce

120 ml/4 fl oz/½ cup water

50 g/2 oz/¼ cup brown sugar

½ head lettuce, shredded

2 tomatoes, sliced

Place the eggs in a saucepan, cover with cold water, bring to the boil and boil for 10 minutes. Drain and cool under running water. Return the eggs to the pan and add the soy sauce, water and sugar. Bring to the boil, cover and simmer for 1 hour. Arrange the lettuce on a serving plate. Quarter the eggs and place on top of the lettuce. Serve garnished with tomatoes.

Tea Eggs

Serves 4–6

6 eggs

10 ml/2 tsp salt

3 China tea bags

45 ml/3 tbsp soy sauce

1 clove star anise, broken apart

Place the eggs in a pan, cover with cold water then bring to a slow boil and simmer for 15 minutes. Remove from the heat and place the eggs in cold water until cool. Leave to stand for 5 minutes. Remove the eggs from the pan and gently crack the shells but do not remove them. Return the eggs to the pan and cover with cold water. Add the remaining ingredients, bring to the boil then simmer for 1½ hours. Cool and remove the shell.

Egg Custard

Serves 4

4 eggs, beaten

375 ml/13 fl oz/1½ cups chicken stock

2.5 ml/½ tsp salt

1 spring onion (scallion), minced

100 g/4 oz peeled prawns, roughly chopped

15 ml/1 tbsp soy sauce

15 ml/1 tbsp groundnut (peanut) oil

Mix all the ingredients except the oil in a deep bowl and stand the bowl in a roasting tin filled with 2.5 cm/1 in of water. Cover and steam for 15 minutes. Heat the oil and pour it over the custard. Cover and steam for a further 15 minutes.

Steamed Eggs

Serves 4

250 ml/8 fl oz/1 cup chicken stock

4 eggs, lightly beaten

15 ml/1 tbsp rice wine or dry sherry

5 ml/1 tsp groundnut (peanut) oil

2.5 ml/½ tsp salt

2.5 ml/½ tsp sugar

2 spring onions (scallions), chopped

15 ml/1 tbsp soy sauce

Beat the eggs lightly with the wine or sherry, oil, salt, sugar and spring onions. Warm the stock then slowly stir it into the egg mixture and pour into a shallow ovenproof dish. Place the dish on a rack in a steamer, cover and steam for about 30 minutes over gently simmering water until the mixture is the consistency of thick custard. Sprinkle with soy sauce before serving.

www.ingramcontent.com/pod-product-compliance
Lightning Source LLC
Chambersburg PA
CBHW071819080526
44589CB00012B/855